The Power of 5

The Power of 5

THE ULTIMATE FORMULA FOR LONGEVITY & REMAINING YOUTHFUL

David Bernstein, M.D.

davidbernsteinmd.com

Published in the United States by Dynamic Learning

Paperback ISBN-13: 9780990708773
ISBN-10: 0990708772
Ebook ISBN 9780990708780
Books are available in quantity for promotional or premium branded corporate use.
For more information on discounts, terms and media requests contact:
Dynamic Learning
Media Department
314 Shore Dr. E. Oldsmar, Florida 34677-3916
Melissa@davidbernsteinmd.com
Visit us at davidbernsteinmd.com or dynamicgrp.com

Books by David Bernstein, M.D.

I've Got Some Good News and Some Bad News...
YOU'RE OLD *Tales of a Geriatrician*
Notes on Living Longer
Senior Driver Dilemmas: Life Saving Strategies

Dedication

It is with extreme gratitude that I dedicate this book to my wife Melissa, the love of my life. She has been by my side throughout the conception, incubation and delivery of this book; without whom there would be blank pages.

Table of Contents

Author's Note

n order to protect the privacy of those mentioned in this book, names and certain identifying characteristics of most patients whose medical histories are described have been changed. Furthermore, all stories were written following HIPAA (Health Portability Act of 1996) compliance guidelines.

Acknowledgements

It would come as no surprise to my readers that I would divide my acknowledgements into five groups, not unlike the five concentric circles I mention in the book.

First and foremost are those are most intimate. My wife Melissa, my partner, best friend, first editor and confidant. She is the most tolerant person I have ever known. every other aspect behind the scenes as well, enabling me to make writing a part of my vocation and avocation. Included in the intimate category is my famlly. My parents, although deceased have always served as shining examples for me to succeed and strive to do the most with my life. My Aunt Flo, who at age 95, is an inspiration as she lives her life following the formula I present in this book. My siblings, Lewis, Nancy and Claire have provided their support and encouragement, providing me a reminder to our roots. The children in my life; who have multiplied through marriages, have played a crucial role for me to set an example for, and in return they have provided their professional expertise in communications and marketing. Each has provided invaluable insight into what it takes to make marketing decisions to enhance my success as an author.

Second, I am grateful to my close inner circle of friends: Jim and Louise Fischer, Craig and Jane Aronoff, Jim and Linda Roberts, David and Susan Herron, Stan and Susan Levy, Albert and Susan Waksman, Steve and Ilene Turker, Michael and Rochelle Brudny, and Jeff and Sue Davis. These friends provided their love and support not only close friends can give, but provided the unconditional assistance for me to strive to complete this publishing project.

Third, I assembled my team that has guided me professionally. It includes editors Carole Green and Kathleen Smith and proof reader Jay Goley. Mari Harper provided social medial support. The Juice Marketing and Design team patiently worked with me on various graphic and design initiatives, including the book cover and graphics used in the book and for presentations. My initial motivation to write came from Martha Murphy and David Fischer.

Forth group include the medical professionals in my community, especially Ben Schaffer who frequently fed me articles that stimulated me to think more about what to include in my writing. Many physician colleagues in my community and hospital have encouraged me along the way: Drs. Rick Schmidt, Robert Davidson, Roberto Bellini, Jon Cobb, Wendy Murphy, Ardeis Scott, David Nicker, and Van Nguyen to name just a few.

A shout out to the Fitness Trainers in my life. I devote the chapter on my approach the Sweat to Rebecca Ibbs, Shannon Crossman, Evangelina DiSpirito, Cindi Bulger and Katherine VanAllan. They were among the most influential and gracious guides, even if I was the only one to show up for an early-morning session.

Furthermore, I have been inspired to include more detailed information about sex and intimacy after I had personal meetings with authors Dr. Ruth Westheimer and Dani Klein Modisett.

And last but not least, the fifth group includes my faithful social media followers to whom I offer my gratitude. They have supported me, sharing enthusiasm for the content of my books.

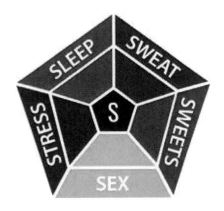

Part I: Introduction to The Power of 5: Disrupting the bonds of longevity

Taking care of your body and brain

Practicing internal medicine and geriatrics for over thirty-five years has given me an opportunity to see successes and failures among my patients. I have discovered five characteristics that usually lead to a happy, healthier, longer life. I've come to think of those five traits by the acronym G R A C E. The letters stand for: Goals, Roots, Attitude, Companionship and Environment. I refer to these again and again during the seminars on aging I present to seniors in my community and nationally. I've had wonderful experiences with my patients, and those interactions have enabled me to visualize this concept as clearly as I do. Furthermore, I believe my community of Clearwater, Florida, reflects what occurs in seniors—and even younger people—not only throughout this country, but also around the world.

In this book I intend to explore and elaborate on how the fifth characteristic of GRACE—Environment—can lead to a happier, healthier, longer life for each of us. Paying attention to Environment can teach us how to work within our own situations to ensure better health for our body and our brain. In other words, paying attention to Environment can teach us to AGE GRACEFULLY®.

My experience includes an office-based practice plus visiting patients in hospital settings, nursing homes and assisted-living facilities. I have had the wonderful opportunity to be chairman of a health systems pharmacy committee, and to function in a twenty-five-year board experience with Jewish Family Services in my community. I've integrated these experiences into my perspectives on aging. I have worked in a collaborative way with my patients to improve the quality of their lives and the length of their days. I've used techniques that are up-to-date and forward thinking, and some that are not necessarily within traditional medical practice. I've had the great pleasure of getting to know my patients to the point they've confided intimate details about their lives. This has enabled me to gain insights into the intricacies of long-standing relationships (some lasting 70 years) and what has led to their longevity. I have developed connections with my patients in a way that helps them to take an active part in preventing and reversing the consequences of their aging. I have realized that it is never too late to make the changes necessary to improve the quality of life—yet I do recommend starting early, or as soon as you are able.

This book will present stories of people from two ends of the spectrum of patients that my colleagues and I see. These anecdotes will illustrate both the good and the bad we see every day. In one way or another, all of these patients motivated me to write this book. In order to protect the privacy of those mentioned within its pages, names and certain identifying characteristics of most patients whose medical histories are described have been changed

Althea was born in a small fishing village in Greece and immigrated to the U.S. as a child. Her father had relatives in New York who helped them get settled and arranged for housing and a good job. Her father was an industrialist and successful, so much so that Althea was able to go to college when she graduated from high school. She earned a bachelor's degree in literature and married shortly thereafter. She always had a positive attitude and took good care of herself. She ate well and exercised almost daily. She had many friends both in the Greek community and in her neighborhood. She raised two intelligent boys and enjoyed her close relationships with family and friends throughout her life.

Widowed at the age of eighty, she became my patient. She had a few minor medical conditions I needed to monitor such as high blood pressure and a thyroid disorder. As a medical patient she was a dream come true. She kept all her appointments, continued to exercise daily, and maintained close relationships with family and friends. As she aged she even developed new friends as many of her older ones died.

At the end of a visit a few years ago I told her about the book I had just published and she said, "Wow, what a great accomplishment. I wish I could do that. I am eighty-five years old and that would be too much for me."

I responded, "If you set your mind to it, I would imagine you could. What would you write about?"

Althea looked at me intently, then said, "I have been thinking of writing about life in the small village where I grew up in Greece. I received my college degree in literature and I have always dreamed about writing my own book."

"Althea," I said, "I know that if you apply yourself, you could do it. You might need to rely on your son to help with the publishing components, but you start writing and I will talk to Jim."

Two years later her book was completed and self-published.

Althea goes on short book tours when she goes north for the summers. She still eats a very healthy diet, and exercises at a fitness center many days a week. She practices yoga three days a week at home. At 92 years old, she has blazed the way for all her friends and family—and me, her doctor.

My second anecdotal example is Ken, who recently reestablished his care in my practice. At his last appointment, eight years ago, he had been a non-compliant patient with diabetes, taking three medications and not following any of my recommendations for diet or exercise. His relationship with his wife was on the rocks and he was drinking ten or more beers a day. He had been diagnosed with sleep apnea and declined treatment due to the inconvenience of the therapy.

He did not return because he and his wife (the family bread winner) no longer had health insurance. During the hiatus, he took none of the three medications I had prescribed and did not eat a healthy diet. He did nothing to improve his diabetes or even check his blood sugar levels. He was not able to work because his obesity had become such an issue. He could not perform his job, his back "gave out," and his feet hurt from his diabetes-related neuropathy. He did not or could not exercise. He was stressed and bickered with his wife when they were not separated. He did not sleep well due to his untreated sleep apnea. The cherry on top was his refusal to address his alcohol abuse; he told me "I'm not an AA person."

I recognized when Ken arrived at my office (as a ticking time bomb) that I was encountering situations that many of my colleagues also see every day. Patients like Ken are part of a major epidemic in this country and around the world. Such ticking time bombs have motivated me to write this book. Without giving too much away at this juncture, I'll say only that Althea's formula for good health and longevity demonstrated her intentions to address five elements that made her extremely healthy at age 93. On the other hand, Ken neglected these five—plus more. This book will detail those five elements and how to incorporate them into your life.

Observations and recommendations in this book are set against a backdrop of disturbing facts and demographics. One troubling set of statistics indicates that the United States healthcare system is the most expensive in the world. Yet, according to a report released by the Commonwealth Fund in 2014 (1), when it comes to health outcomes, Americans fare worse than the general population in eleven similar industrialized nations. This report is one of many that draw similar conclusions.

The Commonwealth Fund report examined the health systems of Australia, Canada, France, Germany, the Netherlands, New Zealand, Norway, Sweden, Switzerland, and the United Kingdom. It found that the United States was last or near last in measures of healthcare access, efficiency and equity. According to the report, the single-payer health system of the United Kingdom ranked first, followed by Switzerland. *The report makes the point that America's lag was largely due to our historic absence of a universal healthcare system.* It's interesting to note that both the U.K. and the U.S. share a low ranking on the "healthy lives" scale that considers infant mortality, healthy life expectancy at age 60, and mortality from preventable conditions such as high blood pressure. The report states that the U.S. system performed best on "effective care"—preventive care efforts such as physicians <u>asking</u> patients to "eat healthy and exercise," and doctors' staff <u>sending</u> patients appointment reminders. (These two items are interesting as they represent data that can be collected from electronic health records for the purpose of evaluating physicians' and their staffs' performance and can be used for compensation purposes.)

On the other hand, the U.S. fared poorly in the Commonwealth Fund report with regards to administrative hassles for doctors and patients, emergency room use, and duplicative medical testing—all part of what is characterized as "efficient care." Personally, I have noticed that it becomes difficult for primary care physicians to obtain relevant clinical information from specialists and hospitals as the data has become voluminous and fragmented. Access to integrated electronic medical records would allow me to provide improved, seamless, coordinated care.

I have also experienced the problem of administrative hassles firsthand; such inefficiency creates tremendous frustration for me as a primary care physician trying to provide cost-effective care to my patients. Recently, one of my patients encountered me outside my office and asked me if my staff had completed the referral for her to have a follow-up appointment with her breast cancer surgeon. The patient has been diagnosed with breast cancer and has an ongoing medical relationship with this physician, yet needed my staff to complete paperwork for her to have a follow-up visit with him. Her surgeon is a very pleasant young man, but I doubt that my patient wanted to visit him for any purpose other than to follow up with her recent breast biopsy.

When I think about the many joys of being a physician that I will miss when I retire, this kind of disruptive hassle to my daily routine won't be one of them.

In evaluating, I am struck by how much we spend in the U.S. for healthcare and how little we get in return.

Graph 1, which follows, illustrates life expectancy and cost. (2) It depicts a significantly lower life expectancy in the U.S against a much higher per capita healthcare expenditure. This is one of the most embarrassing graphs I have seen concerning our system. I personally get a very uneasy feeling when I look at it. I know our healthcare system can and must perform better in this country.

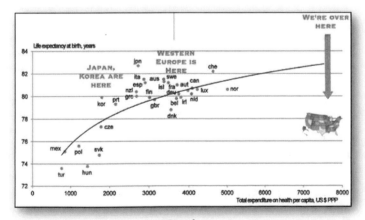

-Graph 1

The information in this book is designed to teach seniors, baby boomers and younger adults how to age in the most gratifying and graceful way. In addition, it will serve to motivate readers to take action and make conscious and intentional choices in order to improve their own health. We all have a certain responsibility. I feel that with a few changes, this graph can look very different in the years ahead.

Over the past hundred years, health in developing countries, particularly the United States, has undergone dramatic changes. As depicted in the graph below, life expectancy has steadily risen.

In the 1930s, average life expectancy was just under sixty years of age. Now, it is over seventy-five. We are living longer but are not necessarily healthier. If the past is any indication of what is likely to happen in our future, we should expect to live even longer, but spend more of that time with a chronic illness or disability.

The greatest improvements in mortality occurred between 1880 and 1950. Graph 2 illustrates life expectancy at birth between 1850 and 1995.

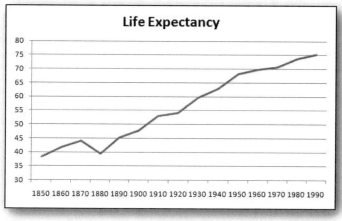

Graph 2

Life expectancy was only 39.4 years in 1880, but increased to 68.2 years by 1950 – an increase of 28.8 years. In the subsequent 40 years, life expectancy went up only a further 7.2 years. (3)

Currently, retirement age in the U.S. is sixty-five and it will increase within the next decade. If we are to retire at that age, we can still expect to live fifteen to twenty additional years. The consequences of this longevity include poor health and disability if we do not take proper care of ourselves before retirement, or if we and our health system run out of money. If we all retire at age sixty-five (an arbitrary age set back in the 1940s, when life expectancy was just over sixty) and we live to eighty-five, we will have a long time to be bored if we haven't prepared, or if we have not remained employed. Either way, attaining better health will prepare us to live a longer, happier, healthier life.

In the 1900s, infectious disease was the leading cause of death. While that danger has decreased, the rate of cancer as a cause of death has tripled. Cancer is now the leading cause of death in the United States. Some of this is related to the improved treatment of infectious disease, leading to higher survival rates, and to improvements in the technologies used for the diagnosis of cancers. Among the cancers, skin, prostate, and breast cancer occur more frequently in both men and women. A bright note: in 1991 the cancer mortality rate started to decrease.

Heart disease still accounts for a large portion of deaths today, as it did in 1900. But major advances in the field of cardiology have made a difference. As an example, I had a conversation recently with a good friend and colleague who has been practicing cardiology in our community for almost as long as I have been practicing geriatrics. We had been attending a social event and, as the program ended, we had a conversation about our recent professional experiences (as professionals often do). My friend told me about some of the new procedures he was introducing into his medical office practice. Though certainly fitting for a cardiologist to perform (especially one with his background and skills), some of them were vascular procedures that had previously been performed only in other settings. I know I was being a bit provocative when I inquired if this evolution occurred because cardiologists had cured all of their patients and had to find something else to do. He laughed, and agreed that great strides had been made. However, he is still busy putting patients on statin medications (used to lower cholesterol levels in the blood) and inserting stents (a tubular support placed temporarily inside a blood vessel, canal, or duct to aid healing or relieve an obstruction) into their coronary arteries when needed.

We laughed and agreed that in fact, statins have made a big difference in the outcomes of patients at risk of dying of heart attacks. And the addition of stents—especially those referred to as "drug eluting stents"—has changed the face of cardiology. Graph 3 below represents the progress made in the field of cardiology since I was born. It shows remarkable changes in our knowledge and understanding of heart conditions. Extraordinary developments between the 1950s and today in medications and technology have altered our cardiac treatments. (4)

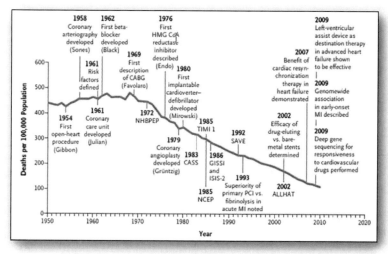

Graph 3

To add to what this graph represents, one of the most important ingredients for living a long and healthy life is listening to one's doctor and taking advantage of what medical science can offer. Medical practitioners do have solutions that can prevent diseases before they occur, and improve outcomes once they develop.

The knowledge I have gleaned, in addition to the observations of thousands of my patients as they have aged over the years, are the key influencers for me to write this book. If it can help even a handful of people to understand and manage their lifestyles and to lead happier, healthier and longer lives, it will have been worth it.

Power of 5 Pointers
Introduction

1. *Living a longer, healthier life is dependent upon adopting healthy habits.*
2. *Unhealthy habits lead to inflammatory conditions and chronic diseases.*
3. *Consequences of inflammation include coronary artery disease, cancer and neurodegenerative diseases.*
4. *Adopting healthy lifestyles can prevent or delay these inflammatory conditions.*
5. *Avoidance of Stress and Sweets and increasing Sweat, Sleep and Sex will enhance longevity.*

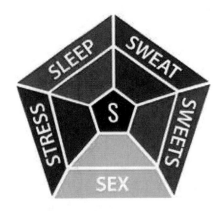

CHAPTER 1

THE POWER OF 5... It is really very simple; we can all do it...

Since my patients have been incredible inspirations for me in both my practice and the writing of this book, I will use many of their stories or composites of several patients' stories to illustrate important factors for my readers to consider.

Fred is another typical example of the kind of "ticking time bombs" that walk into physicians' offices every day. He has been a patient of mine for a number of years. He has enjoyed great success in a 40-year career in the automotive industry, but along the way he paid a significant price in the form of stress. He has amassed moderate wealth, enabling him to eat at some of the finest restaurants in the U.S. and around the world. He loves to travel and particularly enjoys taking his children and grandchildren on lavish vacations.

The banter we share between doctor and patient seems to give him satisfaction, but he follows *none* of the countless recommendations I have given him to improve his health.

His health conditions include obesity, diabetes, hypertension, hypercholesterolemia, coronary artery disease, and atrial fibrillation.

Managing these multiple conditions, while routine for me, has its challenges; having someone who participates so poorly in his own care is astonishing. He has put off until tomorrow every diet or exercise recommendation I've made and seemingly escapes the consequences one would expect, considering his health problems. For me, it seems to defy logic that a man who has amassed the kind of financial resources that enable him to live and enjoy life for a prolonged time is risking it for a big steak and potatoes. At this stage in his life he has enough time on his hands to exercise every day and resources to hire chefs to prepare healthy meals for him, yet he declines.

Recently I have discovered he has sleep apnea—one more condition that puts him at grave risk for heart attack and death. Despite my providing very compelling reasons to wear his CPAP (a breathing device used by patients to correct sleep apnea) he refuses.

As a physician with over thirty years of experience I have tried every professional strategy I know, including sending him to diabetes education, consulting with a dietitian, and recommending a personal trainer. Every time Fred comes back for his quarterly visits, he demonstrates no follow-through or progress to a healthier lifestyle.

Fred's multiple health conditions are common, frequently seen together in the same patient, and make up a substantial segment of the health issues found through the American and Western world. It is for the Freds and Friedas of this world that I have written this book, because I know there is hope.

The components that make up the acronym GRACE. provide a framework for what I have identified as the secrets to live a happier, healthier, longer life: Goals, Roots, Attitude, Connections and Environment. You can read more about them on my blog at **DavidBernsteinMD.com** and in my book *I've Got Some Good News and Some Bad News: YOU'RE OLD!*

With this, my newest book, I will provide important information about modifiable risk factors, or what I refer to as "responding to our **E**nvironment"— the E in GRACE—and what we can do for ourselves to AGE GRACEFULLY®.

After exploring this concept over the years, I have arrived at five easy-to-remember modifiable factors that we can incorporate into our lives to reduce our risk of developing a chronic illness, neurodegenerative diseases of the brain, cancer or premature death from heart disease. I call them "the 5 S's" and together they make up "The Power of 5" formula.

The 5 S's are Sweets, Sweat, Sleep, Stress and Sex

Sweets refers to those sweet and high carbohydrate ingredients within our diet that we need to limit.

Sweat refers to the exercise we need to incorporate into our daily routine.

Sleep refers to the necessity of rejuvenating our brains and our bodies at night.

Stress has been determined as a leading cause of illness, particularly cardiovascular disease and probably cancers.

Sex (which includes aspects of socialization, companionship, intimacy and spirituality) refers to the benefits of having interaction with other people. We can exchange the words sex and spirituality even though they don't have exactly the same meaning, because both relate to relationships between individuals or higher powers.

The relationship between aging/chronic disease and lifestyle

Three main health conditions in our society threaten longevity and lead to most of our chronic diseases. I am referring to cardiovascular disease, neurodegenerative diseases and cancer.

What I discovered as I compiled information for this book and worked on organizing it was that these three major disease groups have similar risks and similar remedies. I knew it innately because I see it every day of my life as a physician. The challenge for me as an author has been to organize the information and present it in an understandable way. In each of the sections of this chapter on cardiovascular disease, neurodegenerative disease and cancer, I will present what I understand to be risks we face in our daily lives and remedies that can help to offset those risks. In the later chapters of the book I will provide more detailed information and actionable steps on how **The Power of 5** can address the risks and improve the odds of avoiding or ameliorating them.

Cardiovascular Disease-Risks
Coronary artery disease in the United States

Study after study has demonstrated that getting sufficient exercise and keeping weight down can have a remarkable effect on health and longevity.

As an example, research suggests that men who adopt five simple lifestyle choices have a far lower risk of cardiovascular events than men who do not. In 1986, researchers from the Harvard School of Public Health began following over 42,000 men in the Health Professionals Follow-up Study. (5) The men had no cardiovascular disease at the time they were enrolled in the study. Researchers then tabulated any cardiovascular events (heart attacks or death) that occurred within this population of men over at least a twenty-five year period. They concluded that had all of the men adopted five healthy lifestyle habits, over sixty percent of the cardiovascular events that occurred within this population would have been prevented.

The five life-saving healthy habits are:

- not smoking
- daily exercise
- prudent eating
- consuming only moderate amounts of alcohol
- maintaining a healthy weight

Only four percent of the men in this study followed all five habits, even though all of the participants were highly educated professional healthcare workers. The men who followed all five habits experienced a full eighty-seven percent reduced risk for cardiovascular disease compared to men who followed none of the healthy habits. Men who adopted two or more of the five healthy habits experienced twenty-seven percent fewer coronary events.

Clinical research has shown again and again that individuals can reduce and control many coronary heart disease (CHD) risk factors with lifestyle changes and medicines. Examples of these controllable risk factors include high blood cholesterol, high blood pressure, and being overweight or obese. Risk factors such as age, gender, and family history cannot be controlled.

To reduce the risk of CHD and heart attack, attempts should be made to control each risk factor. The good news is that many lifestyle changes help control several CHD risk factors at the same time. For example, physical activity may lower blood pressure, help control diabetes and prediabetes, reduce stress, and help control weight. I will address these items later in this book.

Here is an example of a patient and his wife, each with multiple cardiovascular and other risk factors that have yet to be modified. I'll call them Herbert and his wife Edna. I will introduce them now but refer to each of them as their stories relate to other sections in this book. While Fred represents the resistant patients I see every day, as you will see later in this book, Herbert and Edna became more flexible in addressing their lifestyles, as each developed medical conditions requiring attention. I have chosen them as examples of what can happen if you are motivated.

Herbert has been a patient of a colleague of mine for a many years. My colleague had mentioned Herbert to me several times before we met at a party. When we first met, Herbert had a successful career as an engineer and manager and was enjoying his Florida retirement. He was a very studious man; a bit on the obsessive side, he enjoyed spending part of every day surfing the internet to learn about all sorts of things and manage his investment portfolio. He traveled around the world extensively and frequently visited his children and grandchildren who lived out of town. He was slightly overweight; he did not exercise and ate the standard American diet (SAD). His breakfast consisted of orange juice, toast and coffee. He ate sandwiches for lunch. His wife prepared dinner three nights a week, and they went out the other four. Dinner usually consisted of red meat or chicken with a starch.

When we met I could not help but notice that he piled food from the buffet high on his plate, and it included all the high-fat, high-carbohydrate items he could find. The buffet included many previously untasted ethnic foods that, as he tried them, he thoroughly enjoyed. In his own inquisitive fashion, he asked about each before consuming it. He loved the bagels with lox and cream cheese, pickled herring in cream sauce, and, most of all, the cheese blintzes covered with blueberry sauce. He also quickly developed a taste for rugalach. His wife Edna was similarly inquisitive about each item and ate everything she saw as well, obviously savoring every bite. She was substantially heavier.

Herbert knew I worked closely with the host of the party, his physician, so he proceeded to pick my brain during lunch as if he was surfing the internet. He inquired about who each out of town guest was, and then asked about what each item of food he had consumed was made of. When we had finished that line of questioning, he started with the dreaded doctor conversation. "Was there anything healthy about the food served here today? You know, I have normal blood pressure, but my doctor has told me I have metabolic syndrome. I have a total cholesterol which is modestly elevated at 220 but my HDL cholesterol is only 34 and my triglyceride level is 240."

"Are you taking any medication or diet to correct this condition?" I asked (a rhetorical question based on what he had just put on his plate).

"I have declined taking medication to correct my metabolic syndrome so my physician performed an advanced Lipid profile. The test confirmed his concerns about other elements in my bloodstream that put me at risk for a cardiovascular event. We discussed dietary changes over and over, but my wife and I have been resistant to any of the alterations he recommended."

Since we were in a social setting, it seemed inappropriate for me to offer critical remarks or my disapproval. The image in my mind had me shaking my head at what I'd just heard. I knew these two were headed for trouble; Herbert was on a collision course for heart attack, a stroke or premature death. Later in the book, we will have a chance to see what happens to Herbert and Edna.

Cardiovascular Disease—Remedies
Early Prevention
Many lifestyle habits begin during childhood. Thus, parents and families should encourage their children to make heart-healthy choices early in life.

Recommendations include following a healthy diet and being physically active. Just as importantly, following a healthy lifestyle should be a goal for the entire family.

To achieve this goal, learn about key health measures, such as weight, body mass index (BMI), waist circumference, and BMI-for-age percentile. For more information about BMI in adults and children, go to the National Institute of Health (NIH) website and read "Coronary Heart Disease Risk Factors."

It is important for adults to be screened for and, when necessary, treated for elevated blood pressure, blood cholesterol, and blood sugar levels. Once these numbers are known and understood, the patient can work to bring them into a healthy range. Knowledge is power—but making lifestyle changes is a difficult task. Making changes as a family may make it easier for everyone in the household to prevent or control their CHD risk factors.

Healthy Lifestyle Choices
Making healthy lifestyle choices can lower the risk of CHD. For those individuals who already have CHD, a healthy lifestyle may prevent it from getting worse.

Healthy lifestyle is a major focus of this book and will be addressed in greater detail in subsequent chapters. It is the most effective way to fend off the chronic diseases of aging and is the most rewarding strategy to enhance longevity.

A healthy lifestyle, specifically recommended to reduce heart disease, includes:

- following a healthy diet
- being physically active
- maintaining a healthy weight
- smoking cessation
- managing stress

Medicine
Sometimes lifestyle changes alone are not enough to control your blood pressure, cholesterol levels, or other CHD risk factors. In these situations, medicines can be prescribed to:

- lower LDL cholesterol (also known as the bad cholesterol)
- lower blood pressure
- lower blood sugar levels
- prevent blood clots and/or inflammation

Amazing advances have occurred in medications and interventions for the treatment of CHD. On occasion, negative publicity about them is published, but, on the whole, the effectiveness of medications like statins has been proven. I advise consulting reputable sites on the internet and your own physician to gather enough information to make wise decisions.

Patients are encouraged to take medicines as prescribed, not to cut back on the dosage unless a doctor advises it. If side effects or other problems related to any type of medicine develop, patients are encouraged to consult their physician. He or she may be able to provide other options. Continue to follow a heart-healthy lifestyle, even while taking medicines to control your CHD.

Neurodegenerative diseases and the aging brain - Risks

Taking care of your brain is just as important as keeping your body healthy. Dr. Gary Small, geriatric psychiatrist and director of the University of California Los Angeles' Memory and Aging Research Center and Center on Aging at the Semel Institute for Neuroscience and Human Behavior, is confident that brain scientists will make major breakthroughs in the next decade. But it is likely to be a slow and steady process, rather than a single major discovery. Small and his colleagues are now helping people strengthen brain health before memory impairment and other cognitive dysfunction starts to seriously interfere with their daily lives. Medications approved and used to treat Alzheimer's and other kinds of dementia have been lackluster at best; however, research continues in all directions, including looking at the benefits of anti-inflammatory drugs for treating neurodegenerative diseases.

The second of the major chronic conditions threatening longevity is Neurodegenerative diseases. One of the major challenges in addressing neurodegenerative disease compared to cardiovascular diseases and cancers is that the causes are not as clear. Stroke is a major contributor to central nervous system disease, but for the most part, risk for this condition is the same as those previously mentioned in the section on cardiovascular diseases.

Dementia (of which Alzheimer's disease makes up the major portion) and Parkinson's disease are the major central nervous system diseases of aging adults that are believed to be delayed with proper attention to diet and exercise early in life.

I frequently refer to a component of my job and that of my colleagues as being like a detective. I emulate the fictional characters Inspector Clouseau, from the Pink Panther movies, and Lieutenant Colombo, from the TV show *Colombo*. As Clouseau worked to solve a crime he would utter, "Suspect everyone, trust no one."

Lieutenant Colombo would say, "Just one more thing" as he asked one of a number of questions trying to figure out who committed the crime. As I listen and read about crimes in the news I frequently hear about the criminal having a motive and opportunity. When it comes to understanding about the aging process I think about susceptibility and exposure to disease. In the previous section about cardiovascular diseases I consider an individual's susceptibility as their family history or genetic coding and their exposure as the unrestricted diet high in fat and carbohydrates and their inactive, sedentary lifestyle.

When it comes to neurodegenerative diseases the area of susceptibility is not as clear cut. Researchers believe there are genetic causes of Alzheimer's disease, but in a limited number of cases on the order of twenty-five percent. If that is the case, then seventy-five percent of cases are not related to genetics or susceptibility and must therefore have other causes.

Patterns are becoming more recognizable over time. Metabolic factors such as high cholesterol and diabetes are becoming increasingly more suspect, and in a recent study (Flipboard), obesity has been seen as a risk-exposure. Auto-immune conditions where there is a trigger in the body that causes antibodies to attach brain tissue creating inflation and brain cell injury and cell death has been postulated, as well as other inflammatory reactions resulting in the same result.

Stress and depression have been implicated as well as use of certain medications.

Most recently in a report, diphenhydramine (Benadryl) has been implicated as producing symptoms of dementia and possibly inducing the susceptibility to the disease with long-term use. In the past ten years Chronic Traumatic Encephalopathy (CTE) has gained mainstream attention as professional athletes have developed neurodegenerative disease for no reason other than having chronic blows to their heads. Although football players have gained the majority of attention, one of the best known of these athletes was Mohammad Ali. The role of frequent trauma to the head and the resulting concussion (or in some cases without the report of clinical signs of concussion) is now considered a cause of this serious degenerative disease.

I have had my share of experiences as a physician to evaluate individuals with previous brain injuries; they are more common than most of us think. I have seen adults have deterioration in their central nervous system function after a head injury. Even falls with head trauma not initially thought to be of a serious nature have resulted in long-term consequences.

Neurodegenerative diseases—Remedies

Small reveals that lifestyle choices can have an impact on brain health. "We're all on this slippery slope of worsening cognitive ability as we age," he points out. "How rapidly this ability declines depends on genetics and lifestyle...with genetics accounting for about one-third of the probability. But there are things we can do to help sway the odds, and lifestyle choices play a major role and may protect the brain." (6)

Here are four lifestyle changes that can be initiated or enhanced to improve or protect the aging brain:

1. Exercise

A preponderance of scientific evidence points to exercise as the best way to protect the brain. You don't have to become a triathlete. Brisk walking for ninety minutes a week—that's just fifteen minutes a day—has been associated with a lower risk of Alzheimer's disease. And it's not just aerobic or cardio conditioning that has an effect. The data also underscores the benefits of weight or strength training to protect the brain. Recent research even points to a connection between weight loss and improved memory.

2. Stress management

Tests on human subjects who have been injected with the stress hormone cortisol have demonstrated that stress can temporarily impair learning and recall. Depression can also be a risk factor for cognitive impairment. While stress is something we all struggle with, there are things we can do—activities such as tai chi, yoga or meditation.

3. Diet

The Mediterranean diet of olive oil, fish rich in Omega 3 fats, fresh fruits and vegetables that contain antioxidants, and whole grains and nuts can be good for the brain. Avoiding processed foods can also help.

4. Mental exercises

Doing mental exercises can be just as important as doing physical ones. Dr. Small and his team have shown that after a two-week course of brain exercises, one woman's performance on a memory test improved by 200 percent. Other studies have shown similar improvements with such exercises. Although they provide a mental workout, Dr. Small warned that mastery of Sudoku or crossword puzzles may not necessarily translate into sharper memory skills. These exercises are enjoyable but are not novel to the brain of someone who has not already acquired the skill. The ideal is stretching or pushing your brain by learning a new skill. Another way of looking at exercising your brain is partaking in more complex activities such as learning a new or different skill, such as a language or job skill, or taking up a new hobby such as independent publishing (like me).

Cancer-Risks

Cancer in the 21st Century

Pioneering genomic researcher Craig Venter once remarked at a conference, "Human biology is way too complicated as it deals with hundreds of thousands of independent factors. Genes are absolutely not our fate. They can give us useful information about the increased risk of a disease, but in most cases they will not determine the actual cause of the disease, or the actual incidence of somebody getting it. Most biology will come from the complex interaction of all the proteins and cells working with environmental factors, not driven directly by the genetic code." (7)

This statement is very important because we have overemphasized looking to the human genome for solutions to most chronic illnesses, including the diagnosis, prevention and treatment of cancer. Observational studies have indicated that, as we migrate from one country to another, our chances of being diagnosed with most chronic illnesses are determined not by the country we come from, but by the country we migrate to. In addition, studies involving identical twins have suggested that genes are not the source of most chronic illnesses. For instance, between identical twins the concordance for breast cancer has been found to be, at most, twenty percent.

Instead of our genes, it's most likely that our lifestyle and environment account for ninety to ninety-five percent of our most chronic illnesses.

Cancer continues to be a worldwide killer, despite the enormous amount of research and rapid developments in oncology seen during the past decade. According to recent statistics, cancer accounts for about twenty-three percent of the total deaths in the U.S.A. and is the second most common cause of death after heart disease. The rates for heart disease, however, have been steeply decreasing in both older and younger populations in the U.S. from 1975 through 2002. In contrast, over the same period of time, no appreciable differences in death rates for cancer have been observed.

By 2020, the world population is expected to have increased to 7.5 billion people; of this number, approximately fifteen million new cancer cases will be diagnosed, and twelve million cancer patients will die.

Cancer is caused by both internal factors (a five to ten percent contribution from inherited mutations, hormones, or immune conditions) and environmental/acquired factors (a ninety to ninety-five percent contribution from factors such as tobacco, diet, radiation, and infectious organisms). The link between diet and cancer is revealed by the large variation in the rates of specific cancers in various countries, and by the observed changes in the incidence of cancer for people migrating. For example, Asians have been shown to have a twenty-five times lower incidence of prostate cancer and a ten times lower incidence of breast cancer than do residents of Western countries. The rates for these cancers increase substantially when Asians migrate to the West. (8)

The importance of lifestyle factors in the development of cancer was also shown in studies of monozygotic (identical) twins. (9) These studies suggest that only five to ten percent of all cancers appear to be due to an inherited gene defect. Although all cancers are a result of multiple mutations, most of these mutations are due to interaction with the environment.

These conclusions indicate that most cancers are not of a hereditary origin and that lifestyle factors—such as dietary habits, smoking, alcohol consumption, and infections—have a profound influence on their development. Although hereditary factors cannot be modified, lifestyle and environmental factors are potentially modifiable. These observations point to the prevent-ability of cancer. (10), (11), (12), (13)

You'll notice this is a theme that I repeat often in this book.

Avoidable Risks

We know of several avoidable and potentially avoidable risk factors for cancer that can be minimized by making healthier lifestyle choices. Let's look at them individually:

Tobacco

Smoking was identified in 1964 as the primary cause of lung cancer in the U.S. Surgeon General's Advisory Commission Report. Ever since the release of that landmark report, efforts have been ongoing to reduce tobacco use. Tobacco use increases the risk of developing at least fourteen types of cancer, including cancers of the esophagus and mouth. In addition, it accounts for about twenty-five to thirty percent of all deaths from cancer and eighty-seven percent of deaths from lung cancer. Compared with nonsmokers, male smokers are 25 times and female smokers 25.7 times more likely to develop lung cancer. (14) The carcinogenic effects of active smoking are extremely well documented.

Smokeless tobacco

Smokeless tobacco, used for chewing, snuff or dip is a major source of can-cer-causing nitrosamines and is a known cause of human cancer. Using these tobacco products increases the risk of developing cancer of the mouth and throat, esophagus and pancreas. Smokeless tobacco kills fewer people than smoking, but using any form of tobacco harms health and can cause death. (15)

E-cigarettes

Newer and popular alternatives to active smoking, such as electronic cigarettes, also known as vapor or e-cigarettes, and water pipes still contain the addictive chemical nicotine, in addition to other, possibly carcinogenic, chemicals. Among all of the alternative tobacco products, e-cigarettes (battery-operated devices that contain cartridges filled with liquid chemicals that are turned into a vapor or steam to be inhaled) are the least regulated. They have no warning labels and can be sold to people of any age. Many people start using e-cigarettes as a way to quit active smoking, but this strategy has not been approved by the Federal Food and Drug Administration (FDA) and is not necessarily a healthy one.

Secondhand smoke

According to the U.S. Environmental Protection Agency, the U.S. National Toxicology Program, the Surgeon General and the International Agency for Research on Cancer, secondhand smoke is a known human carcinogen. Inhaling secondhand smoke causes lung cancer in nonsmoking adults, with approximately 3,000 lung cancer deaths occurring each year among adult non-smokers in the United States. The U.S. Surgeon General estimates that living with a smoker increases a nonsmoker's chances of developing lung cancer by twenty to thirty percent.

Some research also suggests that secondhand smoke may increase the risk of breast cancer, nasal sinus cavity cancer and nasopharyngeal cancer in adults, and the risk of leukemia, lymphoma and brain tumors in children. (16)

Those who continue to smoke can check with their doctor to learn more about strategies for quitting all forms of tobacco consumption.

Alcohol

The first report on the association between alcohol and an increased risk of esophageal cancer was published in 1910. Since then, a number of studies have revealed that chronic alcohol consumption is a risk factor for cancers of the upper aero-digestive tract, including cancers of the oral cavity, pharynx, hypo-pharynx, larynx, and esophagus, as well as for cancers of the liver, pancreas, mouth, and breast.

The relationship between alcohol and inflammation has also been well established, especially in terms of alcohol-induced inflammation of the liver. How alcohol contributes to carcinogenesis is not fully understood, but the chemical ethanol (which is produced via the fermentation of sugars by yeasts) may play a role.

In the upper aero-digestive tract, twenty-five to sixty-eight percent of cancers are attributable to alcohol, and up to eighty percent of these tumors can be prevented by abstaining from alcohol and smoking. Globally, the fraction of cancer deaths known to be due to alcohol drinking is reported to be 3.5 percent. In the U.S., the number of deaths from cancers known to be related to alcohol consumption could be as low as six percent (as in Utah) or as high as twenty-eight percent (as in Puerto Rico). These numbers vary from country to country (in France this statistic has approached twenty percent in males). (17)

Diet

In 1981, British epidemiologists Richard Doll and Richard Peto (18) estimated that approximately thirty to thirty-five percent of cancer deaths in the U.S. were linked to diet. The extent to which diet contributes to cancer deaths may vary a great deal according to the type of cancer. For example, diet is linked to cancer deaths in as many as seventy percent of colorectal cancer cases. Yet exactly how diet contributes to cancer is not fully understood. Most carcinogens that are ingested—such as nitrates, nitrosamines, pesticides and dioxins—come from food or food additives, or from the cooking process. (19)

Red Meat

Heavy consumption of red meat seems to be a risk factor for several cancers, especially for those of the gastrointestinal tract, but also for colorectal, prostate, bladder, breast, gastric, pancreatic, and oral cancers.

This may be due to the production of the chemical compounds called heterocyclic amines (HCA), during the cooking of meat. The HCAs found in well-done meats and pan drippings are known carcinogens. Charcoal cooking and/or the smoke curing of meat also produces harmful carbon compounds such as pyrolysates and other amino acids (known as "mutagens" for their potential impact at the genetic level), which are thought to be carcinogenic.

The synthetic preservative nitrite, used in some meat products (hotdogs, cold cuts, etc.) is thought to be a powerful carcinogen. Long-term exposure to food additives such as the azo compound dyes found in artificial coloring (such as Disperse Orange 1) has also been associated with carcinogenesis. Furthermore, several studies have shown that the chemical compound bisphenol-a (BPA), used in plastic food containers, can migrate into food and may increase the risk of breast and prostate cancers. BPAs are slowly being removed from the manufacture of plastics and food packaging. (20)

Obesity

According to a 2003 American Cancer Society study (21), obesity has been associated with increased mortality from cancers of the colon, breast (in postmenopausal women), endometrium, kidneys (renal cell), esophagus (adenocarcinoma), stomach, pancreas, prostate, gallbladder and liver. Findings from this study suggest that of all deaths from cancer in the United States, fourteen percent in men and twenty percent in women are attributable to excess weight or obesity.

Worldwide, increased modernization in food production, along with a Westernized diet and a more sedentary lifestyle, has been associated with an increased prevalence of overweight people in many developing countries. (22)

Studies have shown that the factors common to both obesity and cancer include neurochemicals; the abnormal production of hormones such as the insulin-like growth factor 1 (IGF-1) and insulin, the protein leptin; the sex steroids (estrogen, progesterone and testosterone); adiposity; insulin resistance, and inflammation. (23)

Infectious agents *

Worldwide, an estimated 17.8 percent of neoplasms (abnormal tissue growths) are associated with infections. This percentage ranges from less than ten percent in high-income countries to twenty-five percent in some African countries. (24, 25) Some cancers are caused by infections spread by viruses.

> Human papillomavirus, Epstein Barr virus, Kaposi's sarcoma-associated herpes virus, human T-lymphotropic virus 1, Human Immunodeficiency Virus (HIV), Hepatitis B Virus (HBV), and Hepatitis C Virus(HCV) are associated with risks for cervical cancer, anogenital cancer, skin cancer, nasopharyngeal cancer, Burkitt's lymphoma, Hodgkin's lymphoma, Kaposi's sarcoma, adult T-cell leukemia, B-cell lymphoma, and liver cancer.

While the Human T-lymphotropic virus is directly mutagenic, the Hepatitis B and C virus is believed to produce oxidative stress in infected cells and thus to act indirectly through chronic inflammation (26, 27). Other microorganisms, including selected parasites such as Opisthorchis viverrini or Schistosoma haematobium and bacteria such as Helicobacter pylori, may also be involved, acting as cofactors and/or carcinogens (28).

The mechanisms by which infectious agents promote cancer are becoming increasingly evident. Infection-related inflammation is the major risk factor for cancer, and almost all viruses linked to cancer have been shown to activate the inflammatory marker, NF-κB (29)

* Shading of text indicates optional supplemental reading material.

Environmental Factors

Environmental pollution has been linked to various cancers. Culprits include outdoor air pollution from the carbon particles associated with polycyclic aromatic hydrocarbons (PAHs); indoor air pollution from environmental tobacco smoke and its production of volatile organic compounds such as benzene and 1,3-butadiene (which may particularly affect children), formaldehyde and other household contaminants; food pollution from food additives and by carcinogenic contaminants such as nitrates, pesticides, dioxins, and other organo-chlorines; carcinogenic metals and metalloids; pharmaceutical medicines, and cosmetics.

The following types of cancer are linked to environmental exposures:

Bladder
Colon
Gastric
Testicular
Sarcoma and lymphoma
Childhood leukemias, lymphomas, germ cell tumors
Lung cancer

Radiation

According to a 2007 French study, up to ten percent of total cancer cases may be induced by radiation. (30) Cancers induced by radiation include some types of leukemia, lymphoma, thyroid cancers, skin cancers, sarcomas, lung and breast carcinomas. One of the best documented examples of increased risk of cancer after exposure to radiation is the increased incidence of total malignancies observed in Sweden after the population was exposed to radioactive fallout from the Chernobyl nuclear power plant in 1986.

Invisible, hard-to-detect radon and radon decay products in the home and/or in workplaces (such as mines) are the most common sources of exposure to ionizing radiation. The presence of radioactive nuclei from radon, radium, and uranium was found to increase the risk of gastric cancer in rats.

The x-rays used in medical settings for diagnostic or therapeutic purposes are another source of radiation exposure. In fact, the risk of breast cancer from x-rays is highest among girls exposed to chest irradiation at puberty, a time of intense breast development. Other factors associated with radiation-induced cancers in humans are patient age and physiological state, synergistic interactions between radiation and carcinogens, and an individual's genetic susceptibility towards radiation.

Non-ionizing radiation is derived primarily from sunlight. It includes ultraviolet (UV) rays, which are carcinogenic to humans. Exposure to UV radiation is a major risk for various types of skin cancers, including basal cell carcinoma, squamous cell carcinoma and melanoma. Along with UV exposure from natural sunlight, UV exposure from sunbeds for cosmetic tanning may account for the growing incidence of melanoma. Depletion of the ozone layer in the stratosphere can augment the dose-intensity of UVB and UVC, which can further increase the incidence of skin cancer.

Cancer can be prevented with lifestyle change

The fact that only five to ten percent of all cancer cases are due to genetic defects and the remaining ninety to ninety-five percent are due to environment and lifestyle provides major opportunities for preventing cancer.

The following is a list of contributing factors to all cancer deaths in the US:

Tobacco use 25-30%
Infection. 30-35%
Obesity. 15-20%
Other factors 10-15%

Almost ninety percent of patients diagnosed with lung cancer are cigarette smokers. And cigarette smoking combined with alcohol intake can synergistically contribute to tumorigenesis. Similarly, smokeless tobacco is responsible for 400,000 cases of oral cancer worldwide (about four percent of all cancers). Thus avoidance of tobacco products and the minimization of alcohol consumption would likely have a major effect on decreasing cancer incidence.

Inflammation

The analysis of countless studies offers a unifying hypothesis that all lifestyle factors that cause cancer (carcinogenic agents) and all agents that prevent cancer (chemo-preventive agents) are linked through chronic inflammation. The fact that chronic inflammation is closely linked to a tumor-causing pathway, as well as contributing to many other chronic illnesses including cardiac and neurodegenerative disease, is evident from numerous lines of evidence.

Infection

As mentioned earlier, infection by bacteria and viruses is another very prominent cause of various cancers. Vaccines for cervical cancer and liver disease (HCC) should help prevent some of these cancers, and a cleaner environment and modified lifestyle behavior would be even more helpful in preventing infection-caused cancers.

Cancer—Remedies

Diet

Diet, obesity, and metabolic syndrome (the name given to a cluster of risk factors for heart disease, among others) are very much linked to various cancers and may account for as much as thirty to thirty-five percent of cancer deaths. This indicates that a reasonably significant fraction of cancer deaths can be prevented by modifying lifestyle and diet. Extensive research has revealed that a diet that includes certain fruits, vegetables, spices and grains has the potential to prevent cancer. Various phytochemicals (the name given to various biologically active compounds found in plants) have been identified in fruits, vegetables, spices, and grains that exhibit chemo-preventive potential. Numerous studies have shown that a proper diet can help protect against cancer. (31-34)

Below is a description of selected dietary agents and diet-derived phytochemicals that have been studied extensively to determine their role in cancer prevention.

Fruits and Vegetables

The protective role of fruits and vegetables against cancers is now well supported. (35, 36) In 1966, revered American cancer prevention researcher Lee. W. Wattenberg (37) proposed for the first time that the regular consumption of certain constituents in fruits and vegetables might provide protection from cancer.

Fruits and Vegetables

The protective role of fruits and vegetables against cancers that occur in various anatomical sites is now well supported (38, 39). According to a 1997 estimate from the World Cancer Research Fund International, approximately 30–40% of cancer cases worldwide were preventable by feasible dietary means. Several studies have addressed the cancer chemo preventive effects of the active components derived from fruits and vegetables. More than 25,000 different phytochemicals have been identified that may have potential against various cancers.

The following is a short list and descriptions of a few well known phytochemicals found in fruits and vegetables that have been found to have preventive effects.

Carotenoids - Various natural carotenoids present in fruits and vegetables were reported to have anti-inflammatory and anticarcinogenic activity. Lycopene is one of the best known and is a main component in the Mediterranean diet and can account for fifty percent of the carotenoids in human serum. Other carotenoids reported to have anticancer activity include beta-carotene, alpha-carotene, lutein, zeaxanthin, beta-cryptoxanthin, fucoxanthin, astaxanthin, capsanthin, crocetin, and phytoene (40).

Resveratrol - The stilbene resveratrol has been found in fruits such as grapes, peanuts, and berries.

Quercetin - The flavone quercetin (3,3',4',5,7-pentahydroxyflavone), one of the major dietary flavonoids, is found in a broad range of fruits, vegetables, and beverages such as tea and wine.

Silymarin - The flavonoid silymarin is commonly found in the dried fruit of the milk thistle plant Silybum marianum.

Indole-3-carbinol - This flavonoid is present in vegetables such as cabbage, broccoli, brussels sprouts, cauliflower, and daikon artichoke.

Sulforaphane - Sulforaphane (SFN) is an isothiothiocyanate found in cruciferous vegetables such as broccoli

Teas and Spices

Spices are used all over the world to add flavor, taste, and nutritional value to food.

The following is a short list of chemicals found in everyday teas and spices that have potential beneficial effects and cancer protection.

Catechins - Thousands of studies have shown that catechins derived from green and black teas have potential against various cancers.

Curcumin - is another of the most extensively studied compounds isolated from dietary sources for inhibition of inflammation and cancer chemoprevention. In addition to cancer prevention, individuals rely on it to reduce other inflammatory diseases.

Diallyldisulfide - isolated from garlic, inhibits the growth and proliferation of a number of cancer cell lines including colon, breast, glioblastoma, melanoma, and neuroblastoma.

Thymoquinone - found in black cumin considered to have chemotherapeutic and chemoprotective effects

Capsaicin - a component of red chili has been extensively studied. A considerable amount of evidence suggests that it has chemopreventive effects.

Gingerol - is a substance mainly present in the spice ginger; it has diverse pharmacologic effects including antioxidant and anti-inflammatory effects.

Anethole – the principal active component of the spice fennel, has shown anticancer activity.

Diosgenin - a steroidal present in fenugreek, has been shown to suppress inflammation, inhibit proliferation, and induce apoptosis (the death of cells that occurs as a normal and controlled part of an organism's growth or development) in various tumor cells

Eugenol - is one of the active components of cloves. (41)

Wholegrain Foods

Grains form the dietary staple for most cultures, but in Westernized countries most are eaten as refined-grain products. The refining process concentrates the carbohydrate and reduces the amount of other macronutrients, vitamins and minerals because the outer layers of the grain are removed.

Unprocessed whole grains contain chemo-preventive antioxidants. The majority of wholegrain foods we eat are wheat, rice and maize. A secondary group of less popular whole grains are barley, sorghum, millet, rye and oats.

Vitamins

The role of vitamins in cancer chemoprevention is controversial and is being increasingly evaluated. Fruits and vegetables are the primary dietary sources of vitamins except for vitamin D, which is naturally derived from liver and fish oils. Vitamins, especially vitamins C, D, and E, are reported to have cancer chemopreventive activity without the danger of toxicity. It is not clear whether supplementation is the answer or just eating foods rich in these vitamins is where the major benefit is obtained.

Exercise/Physical Activity

Extensive evidence exists to indicate that regular physical exercise may reduce the incidence of various cancers. A sedentary lifestyle has been associated with most chronic illnesses as well as increased risk of cancer of the breast, colon, prostate, and pancreas and of melanoma. (42) The increased risk of breast cancer among sedentary women, due to lack of exercise, has been associated with a higher serum concentration of estradiol, lower concentration of hormone-binding globulin, larger fat masses, and higher serum insulin levels. Physical inactivity can also increase the risk of colon cancer (most likely because of an increase in gastrointestinal (GI) transit time, thereby increasing the duration of contact with potential carcinogens). A sedentary lifestyle may also increase the circulating levels of insulin (promote proliferation of colonic epithelial cells), alter prostaglandin levels, depress the immune function, and modify bile acid metabolism.

I'll explore the larger idea of exercise and physical activity for health and well-being in Chapter 3 – Sweat.

Caloric Restrictions

Fasting is a type of caloric restriction (CR) that is prescribed in most cultures for spiritual or traditional reasons. Dietary restriction, especially CR, is a major modifier in experimental carcinogenesis and is known to significantly decrease the incidence of tumors. The mechanism by which CR reduces the incidence of cancer is not fully understood and more study will be needed in the future.

This overview of the impact that diet and lifestyle choices have on quality of life and health as you age may occasionally sound grim, but it is actually cause for great hope. Why? Because it demonstrates that individuals can take responsibility for and steer their own destiny when it comes to health.

In the chapters to come, I'll show you how.

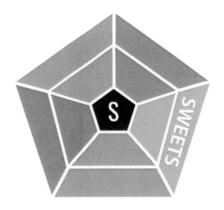

CHAPTER 2

SWEETS... You are what you eat, so don't be Fast, Cheap, Easy or Fake

Throughout my career, my fellow physicians and I have been criticized by almost everyone (including my family members) for not knowing much about nutrition. How can I argue with them? They are correct. The truth is that when I went to medical school, what was then known about "nutrition" pales in comparison to what we know today. In the late 1970s, medical school course work included learning about anatomy, physiology, biochemistry, and other foundational subjects on which to build a strong body of knowledge. These courses were followed by sexy subjects like cardiology, where we learned more dramatically how to save lives. Or obstetrics where we learned how to bring life into the world. For those interested in drama and immediate gratification, surgery was hot, and if you wanted to use your hands, you were lured into gastroenterology. These were areas that seemed to me less engaging, leading to careers associated with great financial rewards, but would possibly be less satisfying for me personally.

When four hours of nutrition study was introduced in our second year, I found it neither sexy, nor hot, nor financially appealing. I recall the instructors' names and what they looked like much more than I can recall anything I learned in class. The material was boring, dry and did not seem relevant to anything else I was interested in. At the time, I did nothing to expand my knowledge in this area. I would come to rue that choice.

However, the climate for the teaching of nutrition is very different today. Every few years a new diet program is introduced. I learn about it, try to see where it could fit into my practice and how I could endorse it or encourage my own patients to follow it. In the last few years, an explosion of good clinical data has really captured my attention. That's because it correlates with my own personal experience and many of the medical conditions I see in my own practice.

Some of my discoveries are:

- the dietary role of fats, especially trans fats
- the explosion in the number of individuals with diabetes and obesity
- the better understanding of the role of carbohydrates and sugars
- the role of exercise and sleep patterns on nutritional state and weight control
- the lack of clear evidence for dietary vitamin supplementation
- the emerging role microbes in the gastrointestinal tract play in nutrition and weight management

Possibly my most important discovery has been that consumers—also known as my patients—often have no clue what to eat. Many of my patients, ranging in age from the mid-fifties up to age ninety, have eaten the same diet for most of their lives and they still cannot distinguish between a protein, a fat or a carbohydrate. This in light of the fact that high-profile, high-protein programs such as the Atkins Diet have been around since the 1970s. That's more than forty years, yet many of my patients still don't get it.

I recently realized just how powerful American breakfast cereal manufacturers and marketers are. The cereal industry has convinced most of the population of the United States to start their day off with dessert (cereal is a very high carbohydrate meal). This same industry is now promoting that we also eat cereal for dinner. If not dessert, what else would you call Cornflakes, Wheaties, Froot Loops, Cap'n Crunch, Cheerios, or even Special K, when they have between thirty and forty grams of sugar and five grams of protein per serving? I am now certain that this marketing phenomenon within our society is driving childhood obesity and contributing to the early onset of diabetes and an increase in heart attacks.

Many patients do not have a clue about what constitutes a healthy diet or the difference in a protein, carbohydrate or a fat. One such patient is Natalie.

Natalie is an example of a typical patient. She is in her late fifties and is overweight, has job and family stresses, high blood pressure and diabetes. She has a college education and raised three children. During one of our visits I inquired about her diet. "Natalie, I have noticed that your test results and weight continue to head in the wrong direction. Please tell me about your diet."

"Doctor", she replied, "you know I have raised my family on a very healthy diet and I know what I am supposed to do. We eat very healthy in our home. We eat very few carbohydrates and high amounts of protein."

"I understand," I said, "but please give me an example of what you consider a high-protein breakfast, lunch, and dinner."

"For breakfast we eat either pancakes with syrup or Raisin Bran. For lunch we usually eat something like tomato soup and a roast beef sandwich, and for dinner most nights we have red meat with a vegetable like corn or green beans and a potato or pasta. I think that is a well-balanced diet low in carbs and high in protein."

I believe Natalie is representative of a vast number of adults who have not had the opportunity to learn the best way to eat or have been so confused by conflicting or complex information from so many sources that they just take the path of least resistance. They choose the least expensive, most convenient option with slight consideration of the health consequence.

Our culture has been led down a path for years. Only now are we becoming aware of the dangers in our diet. Unfortunately, many of my patients have long been under the impression that their diet is healthy and, therefore, remain on the same dietary track. They have no clue how or what to adjust. To further complicate matters, I have found that as we age, change becomes very difficult.

Jarrod has been a patient of mine for many years. That is not his real name, but he will be easily recognizable to most physicians who have certainly had their own patients with a similar history. As he approached his late forties, Jarrod noticed his weight began to increase. He worked hard and dedicated time to his family after hours and on weekends.

But he was totally inattentive to his diet, refusing to make the slightest adjustments to his lifestyle, even as his weight, blood pressure and blood sugar levels rose. His typical response to my recommendations was that I should find a pill to fix his problems. He regularly ate out, including high calorie lunches, and had several alcoholic beverages with and following his dinner. He never exercised and slept poorly. Having two heart attacks and six or seven stents placed in his coronary arteries had no impact on him. He believed he was a caring father to his family, but took absolutely no steps to control his diet. By his late fifties, Jarrod was taking two medications to control his blood pressure and heart ailments, one medication for his cholesterol and two more for his diabetes.

In addition to his hypertension, diabetes, elevated cholesterol and heart disease, he refused to seek counseling for his depression and declined Continuous Positive Airway Pressure (CPAP) therapy for his sleep apnea. It came as no surprise to me when he was fired from his job and his family finally gave up on him. At the time of his employment termination, his monthly medication expense was over $500.

I have to wonder what his life would have been like had he made only a few lifestyle adjustments to correct his poor eating habits.

Obesity

If a person's body weight is at least twenty percent higher than it should be, he or she is considered obese. Obesity has become a global epidemic. It was once only a problem of people living in wealthy nations. Now it impacts countries at all economic levels, bringing with it a wave of poor health and lost productivity. Consider these facts:

- Worldwide the rate of obesity has nearly doubled since 1980, with just over 200 million adult men and just under 300 million adult women now considered obese.
- Obesity rates have been steadily rising in children. In 2010, forty-three million preschool children in the U.S. were overweight or obese, a sixty percent increase since 1990. Folks, pay attention. That's sixty percent more in only twenty years!

- Of all high-income countries, the United States has the highest rates of overweight and obesity, with fully a third of the population currently obese. This rate is projected to rise to around fifty percent by 2030. (43)

Beyond North America, the regions of Europe, South and Central America, Western Pacific, and parts of Africa and Asia also have elevated obesity rates, with only a handful of areas left in the world with consistently low levels of obesity. For many low and middle income countries already struggling in the world economy, obesity takes a particularly high toll—sapping productivity, increasing illness in sole wage earners, and further stretching health systems already burdened with persistent problems of infectious disease and malnutrition. Factors besides a general poor understanding of the proper intake of the components of our diet have led to the increase of obesity rates over the past fifty years. For example, in the U.S., a correlation exists between obesity rates and the increase in consumption of food away from home (FAFH), particularly fast-food consumption. (44)

The worldwide spread of obesity and the resulting increase in rates of chronic disease and other serious conditions threaten health systems, economies, and individual lives. This steady increase will show no sign of slowing without dedicated efforts to combat what I consider to be an epidemic.

Weight Problems Take a Hefty Toll on Body and Mind

Excess weight, especially obesity, diminishes almost every aspect of health, from reproductive and respiratory function to memory and mood. Studies have shown that obesity increases the risk of several debilitating and deadly diseases, including diabetes, heart disease and some cancers, as well as the risk of nonfatal diseases, and conditions such as joint problems and infertility.

It does this through a variety of pathways, some as straightforward as the mechanical stress of carrying extra pounds and some involving complex changes in hormones and metabolism. Obesity generally decreases the quality and length of life, and increases individual, national and global healthcare costs.

The good news, though, is that weight loss can curtail some obesity-related risks. A healthy weight sets the stage for bones, muscles, brain, heart and other components of the body to play their parts smoothly and efficiently for many years. Losing as little as five to ten percent of body weight offers meaningful health benefits to people who are obese, even if they never achieve their "ideal" weight, and even if they begin to lose weight only later in life.

Obesity and Diabetes

The condition most strongly influenced by body weight is type-2 diabetes. In the National Institute of Health's landmark Nurses' Health Study (45), which followed 114,000 middle-age women for fourteen years from 1976, the risk of developing diabetes was ninety-three times higher among women who had a body mass index (BMI) of thirty-five or higher at the start of the study, compared with women with BMIs lower than twenty-two. Weight gain during adulthood also increased diabetes risk, even among women with BMIs in the healthy range. (46) The Health Professionals Follow-Up Study found a similar association in men. (47)

Fat cells—especially those stored around the waist—secrete hormones and other substances that cause inflammation. Although inflammation is an essential component of the immune system and part of the healing process, inappropriate inflammation can produce a variety of health problems. Inflammation can make the body less responsive to insulin and alter the way the body metabolizes fats and carbohydrates, resulting in higher blood sugar levels and, eventually, to diabetes and its many complications. Several large trials have shown that even moderate weight loss can prevent or delay the start of diabetes in people who are at high risk. (48)

As we return to the health saga of Herbert and Edna, Herbert's health scare was the first of the events to happen. Shortly after returning from his morning walk, he said, "I developed a mild discomfort in my left shoulder. I thought it was just a mild sprain and waited until after dinner. It did not get any better so I went to the ER. In the ER they did a bunch of tests including an EKG and enzymes test. In all it revealed I was suffering a heart attack. Within minutes, a cardiologist was at my bedside and thirty-five minutes later I had two stents placed in my heart. They tell me one was in the "widow-maker artery. I guess I got lucky, Doc."

Herbert was discharged one day after the stents were placed and was given a prescription for medication to improve his cholesterol and a copy of a diet to follow to reduce his cardiovascular risk. One would think that having a heart attack would be enough motivation to make lifestyle changes, but Herbert was not so motivated. When a stent can avert a heart attack so quickly, some of the motivation is lost. Herein lies another one of the problems in our healthcare system and patients' lack of accountability.

Obesity and Metabolic syndrome

Another major consequence of obesity (and a main factor contributing to the problems of my patient, Jarrod, mentioned above) is one that many primary care physicians see multiple times a day. It is usually known as metabolic syndrome. The term "metabolic" refers to the biochemical processes involved in the body's normal functioning. Other names for metabolic syndrome include dysmetabolic syndrome, insulin resistance syndrome, obesity syndrome or syndrome X.

All of these names refer to the same group of risk factors for heart disease and other health problems, such as diabetes and stroke. Metabolic syndrome is becoming more common due to a rise in obesity rates among adults and may, in the future, overtake smoking as the leading risk factor for heart disease. Individuals with metabolic syndrome are at risk for coronary heart disease (CAD), the condition caused when the waxy substance known as plaque builds up inside the coronary (heart) arteries. Plaque hardens and narrows the arteries, reducing blood flow to the heart muscle. This can lead to chest pain, a heart attack (myocardial infarction), heart damage, or even death. In addition, we also know that the soft variety of this plaque, which is due to the inflammatory process mentioned earlier, is prone to rupture resulting in attraction of platelets and then complete closure of an artery. This is an even more common cause of heart attacks.

The following five conditions can be indicative of metabolic syndrome. The diagnosis is made when testing has determined that an individual has at least three of the following risk factors.

Excess fat in the stomach area is a greater risk factor for heart disease than excess fat in other parts of the body, such as on the hips. A waist measurement of thirty-five inches or more for women or forty inches or more for men is considered a metabolic risk factor.

Triglycerides are a type of fat found in your blood. **A triglyceride level of 150 milligrams per deciliter (mg/dL) or higher**, or being on medication to treat high triglycerides is considered a metabolic risk factor.

HDL Cholesterol (high density lipoprotein) is sometimes called "good" cholesterol because it helps remove "bad" or LDL cholesterol from your arteries. A low HDL cholesterol level of less than 50 mg/dL for women and less than 40 mg/dL for men raises an individual's risk for heart disease. **A low HDL cholesterol level is considered a metabolic risk factor, as is being on medicine to treat it.**

If **blood pressure** rises and stays high over time, it can damage your heart and lead to plaque buildup. A blood pressure of 130/85 mmHg (millimeters of mercury) or higher (or being on medicine to treat high blood pressure) is a metabolic risk factor. If only one of the two blood pressure numbers is high, risk for metabolic syndrome persists.

Mildly high fasting blood sugar levels may be an early sign of diabetes. A normal fasting blood sugar level is less than 100 mg/dL. A fasting blood sugar level between 100 and 125 mg/dL is considered pre-diabetes. A fasting blood sugar level of 126 mg/dL or higher is considered diabetes. **A fasting blood sugar level of 100 mg/dL or higher (or being on medication to treat high blood sugar) is considered a metabolic risk factor.**

An individual's risk for heart disease, diabetes and stroke increases with the number of metabolic risk factors. In general, a person who has metabolic syndrome is **twice** as likely to develop heart disease and **five** times as likely to develop diabetes as someone who doesn't have metabolic syndrome.

The risk of having metabolic syndrome is closely linked to overweight and obesity and a lack of physical activity. Insulin resistance—a condition in which the body can't use its insulin properly—also increases the risk for metabolic syndrome. Insulin is a hormone that helps move blood sugar into cells, where it's used for energy. Insulin resistance can lead to high blood sugar levels, and it's closely linked to overweight and obesity. Genetics (ethnicity and family history) and older age are other factors that may play a role in causing metabolic syndrome.

Happily, lifestyle changes can prevent or delay metabolic syndrome. But achieving a healthy lifestyle requires a **lifelong** commitment. Successfully controlling metabolic syndrome requires long-term effort and teamwork with your healthcare providers.

Other medical conditions that appear to be associated with metabolic syndrome include: a fatty liver (excess triglycerides and other fats accumulating in the liver), polycystic ovarian syndrome (a tendency to develop cysts on the ovaries), gallstones and breathing problems during sleep (such as sleep apnea).

Some individuals are at risk for metabolic syndrome because they take certain medicines that cause weight gain or changes in blood pressure, blood cholesterol or blood sugar levels. These medicines most often are used to treat inflammation, allergies, HIV, and depression and other types of mental illness.

Healthy lifestyle changes are the first line of treatment for metabolic syndrome. Lifestyle changes can include losing weight, being physically active, following a heart healthy diet, and quitting smoking.

If lifestyle changes aren't enough, physicians may prescribe medicines. Medicines are used to treat and control risk factors such as high blood pressure, high triglycerides, low HDL cholesterol and high blood sugar.

"Blood-thinning" medicines such as aspirin (which inhibit platelet activity), also may be used to reduce the risk of blood clots, a condition that often occurs with metabolic syndrome.

Obesity and Cardiovascular Disease

Body weight is also directly associated with various cardiovascular risk factors. As BMI increases, so do blood pressure, LDL or "bad" cholesterol, triglycerides, blood sugar and inflammation. These changes translate into increased risk for coronary heart disease, stroke and cardiovascular death. (49)

As noted above; coronary artery disease (CAD) is the ongoing accumulation of fat and cholesterol-laden plaque in the blood vessels supplying the heart. When these vessels become sufficiently narrowed, less oxygen and nutrients reach the heart, causing symptoms of chest pains or shortness of breath. These vessels can become abruptly blocked or obstructed causing a myocardial infarction or what is commonly known as a heart attack. A stroke occurs via a similar progression as CAD. There is a buildup of plaque, in an event similar to what happens in the heart, and one of the main blood vessels supplying the brain becomes occluded, resulting in infarction or the death of brain tissue. When an individual dies from either a heart attack or a stroke, we regard this as a cardiovascular death.

Consider the following studies:

- A group of investigators conducted a meta-analysis of twenty-one long-term studies that followed more than 300,000 participants for an average of sixteen years. Study participants who were overweight had a thirty-two percent higher risk of developing CAD, compared with participants who were at a normal weight; those who were obese had an eighty-one percent higher risk. (50)
- In an analysis of twenty-five observational studies that included 390,000 men and women of several racial and ethnic groups, obesity was significantly associated with cardiovascular disease and death from CAD. There was favorable news in that weight loss of five to ten percent of body weight could lower blood pressure, LDL cholesterol, and triglycerides, and therefore improve other cardiovascular risk factors. (51)
- Stroke and CAD share many of the same disease processes and risk factors. Studies have demonstrated a direct association between excess weight and stroke risk. In one meta-analysis of twenty-five separate studies, data showed that being overweight increased the risk of ischemic stroke by twenty-two percent, and obesity increased it by sixty-four percent. (52)

Herbert had been feeling well and did start to exercise by walking. He even delayed his daily web surfing to start a workout routine at a local fitness center. He had not reached the point of making the diet changes he needed until something happened to his wife. Edna had an abnormal mammogram. After weeks of testing and waiting for results, she was diagnosed with breast cancer. Herbert began to heavily research the impact that diet, obesity and exercise had on the development and recovery from cancer. It was at that point the Herbert and Edna made lifestyle changes in their household.

Obesity and Cancer

The association between obesity and cancer is not as clear cut as that for diabetes and cardiovascular disease. This is due in part to the fact that cancer is not a single disease but a collection of individual diseases. In data, released in 2007, an expert panel assembled by the World Cancer Research Fund and the American Institute for Cancer Research concluded there was convincing evidence of an association between obesity and cancers of the esophagus, pancreas, colon and rectum, breast, endometrium, and kidney, and a probable association between obesity and gallbladder cancer. (53) Abdominal obesity and weight gain during adulthood were also linked with several cancers. A subsequent review confirmed direct associations between obesity and cancers of the breast, colon and rectum, endometrium, esophagus, kidney, ovary and pancreas. (54) The Nurses' Health Study has found some favorable results: for overweight women who have never used hormone replacement therapy, losing weight after menopause—and keeping it off—cuts their risk of post-menopausal breast cancer in half. (55)

Obesity, Depression, and Quality of Life

The observations have noted high rates of obesity and depression with cardiovascular disease. This has led investigators to explore the relationship between weight and mood. Analysis of cross-sectional studies found that people who were obese were more likely to have depression than people with healthy weights. (56) Newer evidence revealed that the relationship between obesity and depression may be a two-way street. Long-term studies that followed 58,000 participants for up to twenty-eight years found that people who were obese at the start of the study had a fifty-five percent higher risk of developing depression by the end of the follow-up period, and people who had depression at the start of the study had a fifty-eight percent higher risk of becoming obese.(57) It has been suggested that the link between obesity and depression has not yet been definitively identified. Possible mechanisms include activation of inflammation, changes in the hypothalamic–pituitary–adrenal axis, insulin resistance, and social or cultural factors.

Obesity and Lung Function/Respiratory Disease

Excess weight impairs respiratory function via mechanical and metabolic pathways. The accumulation of abdominal fat, for example, may limit the descent of the diaphragm, and in turn, lung expansion, while the accumulation of fat in the viscera covering the ribcage can reduce the flexibility of the chest wall, sap respiratory muscle strength and narrow airways in the lungs.

Obesity is also a major contributor to obstructive sleep apnea (OSA), which is estimated to affect approximately one in five adults. This condition is associated with daytime sleepiness, accidents, hypertension, cardiovascular disease, and premature mortality. Between fifty percent and seventy-five percent of individuals with OSA are obese. (58) Clinical studies and observation from sleep experts suggest that modest weight loss can be helpful when treating sleep apnea.

Obesity, Memory, and Cognitive Function
Alzheimer's disease and dementia are ever-growing concerns in an era when enjoying a long life span has become more common. In the United States, these diseases affect more than 7.5 million people, most of them over age sixty-five. (59) It is well accepted that body weight is a potentially modifiable risk factor for both Alzheimer's disease and dementia. One study has demonstrated an unusual and unexpected association between BMI and Alzheimer's disease. Compared with being within the normal weight range, being underweight was associated with a thirty-six percent higher risk of Alzheimer's disease, while being obese was associated with a forty-two percent higher risk. (60) The associations were even stronger in studies with longer follow-up.

Obesity and Musculoskeletal Disorders
Excess weight places mechanical and metabolic strains on bones, muscles, and joints. In the United States, an estimated forty-six million adults (about one in five) report doctor-diagnosed arthritis. (61) Osteoarthritis of the knee and hip are both associated with obesity, and obese patients account for one-third of all joint replacement operations. Obesity also increases the risk of back pain, lower limb pain, and disability due to musculoskeletal stress.

Obesity and Sexual Dysfunction
It has been well established that obesity may have an effect on sexual function. Numerous sources reveal an increase in erectile dysfunction with increasing BMI. In addition, weight loss has been found to improve this dysfunction. The effect of obesity on women is less certain. In one study on sexual function

there was a strong correlation between increasing BMI and problems with arousal, lubrication, orgasm and satisfaction. (62)

Lifestyle Changes and Obesity Prevention

Just now medical literature has confirmed that obesity harms virtually every aspect of health, shortening life, contributing to chronic conditions such as diabetes and cardiovascular disease, and interfering with sexual function, breathing, mood and social interactions.. Obesity and the health risks it contributes to aren't necessarily permanent conditions. Diet, exercise, medications, and even surgery can lead to weight loss. However, I have observed as a physician and in my own experiences that it is much, much harder to lose weight than it is to gain it. Prevention of obesity, beginning at an early age and extending across the life span, could vastly improve individual and public health, reduce suffering and save billions of dollars each year in healthcare costs.

In the second half of this chapter and in each of the subsequent chapters of this book, I will describe in detail how to go about making healthier lifestyle choices for longevity. But because some of the statistics I've been citing are so dismal, here are a few highlights of my Power of 5 formula to give you hope and get you thinking:

Set realistic short- and long-term goals when you begin to make healthy lifestyle changes. Work closely with your doctor and seek regular medical care.

For those individuals who have metabolic syndrome and are overweight or obese, their doctors will likely recommend weight loss. He or she can help create a weight-loss plan and set realistic goals. Attempting to make changes to lower your BMI to less than twenty-five would have favorable benefits. One way to accomplish this is to calculate BMI using the National Heart, Lung, and Blood Institute's (NHLBI's) online calculator** [https://www.nhlbi.nih.gov/health/educational/lose_wt/bmitools.htm], or in consultation with a health-care provider.

A heart-healthy diet is an important part of a healthy lifestyle. It should include a variety of vegetables and fruits, either fresh, canned, frozen or dried. A good rule is to try to fill at least half of your plate with vegetables and fruits.

A healthy diet also includes whole grains, fat-free or low-fat dairy products, and protein foods such as lean meats, poultry without skin, seafood, processed soy products, nuts, seeds, beans, and peas. In part two of this book there will be illustrations of what your plate should look like at each meal.

Choose and prepare foods with little sodium (salt). Too much salt can raise an individual's risk for high blood pressure. Studies show that following programs such as the popular DASH diet** (DASH is an acronym for Dietary Approaches to Stop Hypertension) [http://dashdiet.org] can lower blood pressure.

Adjusting a diet to avoid foods and drinks that are high in added sugars is important as well. For example, drink water instead of sugary drinks like soda and many juices.

Limit the amount of solid fats and refined grains eaten. Solid fats are saturated fat and trans fatty acids such as butter and shortening. Refined grains come from over-processing whole grains, resulting in a loss of nutrients such as dietary fiber.

For individuals who drink alcohol, it should be done in moderation. Too much alcohol can raise blood pressure and triglyceride levels. Alcohol also adds extra calories, which can cause weight gain.

Aim for a healthy weight by staying within daily calorie needs. Balance the calories taken in from food and drinks with the calories used while doing physical activity. There are many online programs and smart-phone apps that are extremely helpful in calculating daily caloric requirements. One's daily requirements change as weight fluctuates. In addition, these programs will encourage keeping a log or diary of daily food intake, which is another proven way to control and reduce body weight. Of the many apps I am aware of, two are *Lose It*** and *Fitbit***.

Physical activity can help keep your heart and lungs healthy. Even modest amounts of physical activity are good for your health. The more active you are, the more you'll benefit. Before starting any kind of exercise program or new physical activity, however, I encourage a discussion with a physician about the types and amounts of physical activity.

For individuals who smoke, quit. Smoking can raise one's risk for heart disease and heart attack and worsen other heart disease risk factors. I encourage

---

** Resource Section in back of book

talking to a doctor about programs and products that can help quit smoking. Also, try to avoid secondhand smoke.

I encourage those who have trouble quitting smoking on their own join a support group or class at a local hospital, at work or through a community organization.

If lifestyle changes aren't enough, physicians may prescribe medicines to help control risk factors. Medicines such as statins can help treat unhealthy cholesterol levels. High blood pressure is treated with diuretics or angiotensin-converting enzyme (ACE) inhibitors that dilate blood vessels and increase blood flow. High blood sugar is treated with oral medicines such as metformin, insulin injections, or both. Low-dose aspirin can help reduce the risk of blood clots, especially for people whose risk of heart disease is high.

It seems amply evident that diet can play a huge role in promoting health and preventing disease. In this chapter on "**Sweets**" I've explored the science behind poor food choices and how they impact bodily functions. At the end of this book, I have compiled tips on nutrition and guidelines for making healthier dietary choices. I've even provided a series of heart- friendly recipes to kickstart your journey to a better, healthier life.

The Power of 5 is all about taking back power and responsibility for the quality of your life. I'm on your side, as are many primary care physicians and medical specialists across the country. Let's work together to reduce rates of obesity and its negative impact on every aspect of life in the 21st century.

S is for Sweets - Formula
The Outrageous Benefits of Eating Well

After my first book, *I've Got Good News and Bad News – You're OLD!* was published in 2014, it became apparent to me that it was being lumped in with all the self-help books dealing with diet, exercise and nutrition. Imagine the competition to get into a Top Ten listing, knowing that the entire world is looking for that one special diet book. Don't get me wrong; some excellent self-help books have come to the market. In fact, I have reviewed many in preparation for writing this one. But I have also endeavored to avoid the word "diet" when I write about the lifestyle changes needed in order to AGE GRACEFULLY® and avoid the chronic diseases I've mentioned earlier in this book. I have listened to advisors who mentioned the seven-day this and thirty-day that diet, or the famous-celebrity-turned-diet-expert touting the best way to look thinner in ten days. My recommendations are geared not only toward weight loss, but to weight loss as a likely byproduct of lifestyle change.

> Recently, I had a very health-conscious patient named Nora visit my office. For several years I have been successfully treating her high blood pressure and high cholesterol with medication. She is very satisfied and feels that she eats a very healthy diet. We discussed her meal plan and the challenges she faces feeding her picky family. Her husband, Tim, who is also a patient, who takes medication to reduce his triglycerides. He is content with his regimen, but Nora tells me she has to prepare two different meals each night because Tim will not eat vegetables. He eats only meat and potatoes. I find this ridiculous. The man is in his late fifties and has still not woken up to the fact that his diet is the main reason he is taking medication. He wants to live a long and healthy life, but seems unwilling to make the lifestyle changes needed to help make that happen.

Since I am not a dietician or trained nutritionist I can only make suggestions about what constitutes the healthiest lifestyle. My ideas are based on my research and observations about what might enhance a person's chances of living a long and healthy life. I have purposely avoided the word "diet" to describe the changes I recommend about food. I prefer the word "lifestyle," because it suggests the ways in which you will change forever. People "go on" diets and then "go off" diets. I am promoting a lifestyle that will work, will be energizing, and is easy enough to do.

There will be a lot of vegetables. I hope you like them. As a small reminder: when we first encounter Adam and Eve in the Bible, they are in "The **Garden** of Eden." I was not there, but I bet they survived on fruits and vegetables.

The Problem with Modern Food Habits

Food with high concentrations of carbohydrates, especially those with high sugar content, stimulate the release of insulin and other chemicals that lead to inflammation and suppression of the immune system. This can lead to a higher risk of vascular disease and cancer.

It is also important to recognize that worldwide, and particularly in the United States, in the past thirty years meal portion sizes have increased dramatically. One very important feature of the lifestyle changes I recommend is the reduction or resizing of meals and some awareness of the total number of calories certain foods contain. The truth is that with the changes I advise, calorie counting becomes much less of an issue. Nonetheless, it is worth being aware of caloric intake. Most of the vegetables I recommend eating have fewer calories than most of what I would consider the unhealthy foods many people eat today. It is also well documented how much portion sizes have increased in restaurants. Considerable data in various studies support this view, and I have alluded to it in the first part of this book. This does not mean your new lifestyle will not allow you to eat out; it just means you need to become selective and not fall into the traps that restaurateurs have set for you.

My own research, based on a review of medical literature and many patient encounters, shows that an eating style similar to those who live in countries bordering the Mediterranean is the healthiest, easiest, most affordable, portable, and flexible. This eating style is packed with fresh fruits and vegetables, which are plentiful and readily available in most developed countries. Looking at other kinds of diets for comparison, all have high concentrations of the proper mix of fruits and vegetables, so there is nothing objectionable there (except to my sister Nancy). I will point out that there are certain vegetables that I consider taboo—the ones that are high in starchy carbohydrates—such as potatoes, and root vegetables. Fruits with high concentrations of sugar are also to be avoided or eliminated.

Major Food Groups

The first major element in my recommendation for following a healthier diet is an increased consumption of vegetables. **The Power of 5** Formula contains at least forty percent vegetables. Falling into that broad general category are vegetables that can be eaten raw or cooked. Readily available examples are lettuce, tomatoes, celery, cucumber, and zucchini. The list goes on.

The second major component of **The Power of 5** Formula is the eating program which includes healthier low-fat protein. I prefer fish or seafood, as they are lower in calories and healthier to eat. Healthy protein should comprise approximately twenty percent of your meal. The protein portion size equates to four to eight ounces (approximately the size of the palm of your hand.).

The third aspect of **The Power of 5** Formula for eating well includes foods that contain healthy fat. Avocados and nuts fall in this category. The formula allocates twenty percent of the meal to this food group.

The next grouping of food contains healthy carbohydrates. These are foods such as legumes (things like kidney beans, chickpeas and lentils). I avoid most carbohydrates, especially grains, but feel that a few exceptions are okay.

Earlier in this chapter I expressed my belief that Madison Avenue marketers have brainwashed our population into thinking that our day should start with breakfast cereal composed mostly of highly processed wheat and laden with processed sugar. In addition, I believe that today's wheat has been genetically modified. It is not the same as it was many years ago when I was growing up. It is no longer the same grain that was used to make the bread I was brought up on in the 1950s and 1960s.

Since our bodies need energy all day long to keep them functioning, it is important to provide them with nutrition all day long. I suggest that the three major meals of the day be appropriate in size to meet your demands. In addition, two low-calorie, high-protein snacks may be consumed. I find that low-carbohydrate protein bars or similar shakes are convenient and not particularly disruptive to one's daily routine. I will reiterate: In order for an individual to adopt a revised lifestyle such as **The Power of 5** Formula, it must be simple, portable, adaptable, and tasty. Check out the easy recipes from **The Power of 5** test kitchen in part two of this book.

The Upside of Snacking

Snacks are a fact of North American culture, but they are often consumed in unhealthy quantities. **The Power of 5** lifestyle and eating plan includes two daily snacks in between meals. With care, snacking can add nutritional value and balance out energy levels throughout the day. Here are a few suggestions for healthy snacks to include in your weekly menu planning and shopping routine.

- Protein shakes—these can be made with yogurt and fruit with the addition of vitamin or protein supplements.

- Crudité vegetables—raw, peeled vegetables such as celery, carrots or cucumber. Eat with a small amount of low-fat dip made from yogurt or chickpea hummus.
- Fresh fruits—berries, tangerines or apples, or dried fruits such as raisins or apricots in limited quantities.
- Healthy nuts—almonds, cashews and pistachios

What to do about dining out

It is extremely important to our success—especially when starting out with this new lifestyle plan—to avoid temptation. So choosing an appropriate place to enjoy a healthy meal out is the best place to start. Choose restaurants where you know the menu and trust that staff won't obnoxiously push unnecessary appetizers and unhealthy food selections. Choose a restaurant that offers lots of choice in salads and vegetables. Consider a Mediterranean or vegetarian restaurant; both will have healthy and delicious options on the menu. Here are a few tips to help make your dinner out memorable for the enjoyment of good food and company, rather than for the guilt of having messed up.

- Water is your friend.
  Hydrate before and upon arrival at your chosen restaurant (this does *not* mean alcohol). I have read that some of us have bodies that confuse hunger with the need to hydrate. Whether or not you are actually hungry, it is a good idea to enter the restaurant well hydrated, to avoid the potential of being overwhelmed with feelings of dehydration masked as hunger.
- Review menus beforehand if it's possible.
  Most restaurants post their menus online, or, at the very least, outside the front door. If not, ask to see a menu before deciding to eat at a restaurant that is new to you. Don't allow yourself to be surprised or confused into having fewer choices than you need.
- See to it that your choice of restaurant includes salad options and that high-calorie, sugar-enhanced dressings can be omitted and you can have a tablespoon of olive oil and vinegar instead.

- Avoid buffets—just say no!
  For many of us there is a psychological issue when dining at a buffet. We demand to get our money's worth. As a result, we go overboard and not only consume the unhealthy items, but too many of them. Personally, with rare exceptions, I never see dining buffet set-ups that offer mainly healthy food.
- Avoid the bread and rolls.
  The lifestyle I recommend asks you to eliminate most grains, especially bread, so the first thing to do is to tell your waiter not to serve the bread basket.
- Split an appetizer, salad, dessert, or even an entire meal, with a dining companion.

Having a supportive partner is a great way to make lifestyle changes. As I indicated previously, most eating establishments provide far more calories for each meal than most people need for a single serving. Sometimes, restaurant meals could easily feed three. Your partner should be agreeable and willing to compromise on selections. Even if you have to alternate who makes the choice from meal to meal, this habit delivers great payoffs. Not the least of which is that you will save a few bucks in the process.

Above all, have fun by enjoying your meal and your company. Being prepared takes away any pre-meal ordering uncertainty.

Eating and Social Occasions

Much of what has been listed in the above section applies to all kinds of events including family gatherings, weddings and other special events, picnics, sporting events, and tailgate parties. But it bears repetition.

Avoid bread.

It is just too easy to pick up a sandwich or sub and hold it in your hand at one of these events. Before you even know it, you have eaten a hamburger or hot dog, and are looking for more. Consider lettuce wraps as an alternative to conventional sandwiches. By avoiding bread, you make a conscious effort to follow the lifestyle changes I advise (or prescribe). If you are the host or someone has asked you to bring an item, don't be shy; bring something that you and hopefully others will enjoy. Lettuce wraps are a great choice, especially stuffed with healthy, high-protein ingredients such as chicken breast, sliced turkey, fish, veggies, or even tofu.

Pack your own sensible meal with plenty of fresh vegetables.

It is certainly reasonable to bring your own food to many of these kinds of events. My wife and I always carry a small sack of healthy snacks when we attend professional baseball games. We end up impressing the onlookers, and save a bundle by not buying the expensive and grossly unhealthy food served at the stadium.

Salads

Based on everything I have recommended so far, it goes without saying that you should gravitate to healthy salads. But watch out for unhealthy additives like sugar and other carbohydrates such as croutons. Salad dressing can be full of fats and preservatives, so ask what is in the dressing.

Veggies, veggies, veggies

They're easy to hold in your hand and eat as many as you want. Just avoid dipping them into something laden with fat, carbs and sugar.

Sensible fruit

You can overdo it with fruit, but, for the most part, as long as you maintain some level of control, they are a much better alternative to brownies or ice cream.

Remain hydrated.

Drink plain water, as it will reduce the possibility of your brain mistaking dehydration for hunger.

Bring your own healthy shake or smoothie. Arriving well-nourished reduces the probability of overeating the minute you sit down, and during the entire event.

Beer and alcohol can have negative effects and offset many of the healthy gains you have made. Avoid them, but if you cannot, enjoy them in moderation.

Fast Food and FAFH

In spite of the guidelines I have provided above, eating fast food or food eaten away from home (FAFH) is generally tricky and not recommended. Fast-food establishments are in the business of getting food to the customer fast. There is no guarantee that it will be healthy because the food contains inexpensive ingredients and is made (or pre-made) and served rapidly. Some exceptions have splashed onto the scene, with a handful of entrepreneurs taking a dive into the business of preparing healthy meals for people on the go.

One of my patients, Dennis, who has been struggling with his weight, diabetes and high cholesterol, related the following story to me. He and his wife planned a very busy summer. They planned a cross-country bus tour lasting four weeks. During that time renovations were to be performed in their kitchen and bathrooms. They hired a great contractor and an individual to watch over the project to be certain it progressed on time. The project proceeded according to schedule as he and his wife ate all their meals (three daily) at restaurants or buffets. For reasons I've already described, they were not able to control what was put before them. They had different meal preferences so rarely split a meal. Once home, they noticed a modest but still notable weight increase. It was a struggle for both. As they planned to start using their new kitchen, they experienced a setback. A pipe in the newly installed refrigerator leaked the day before they were to move back in, destroying the hardwood floors and prompting an additional six weeks of living away from their home. This problem subjected them to more meals eaten away from home.

What I found disturbing in this real-life situation was the absence of a strategy or clear plan to address the temptation to make bad choices. I also felt bad that they did not compromise and split any of their meals.

Here are a few more FAFH situations that can trigger poor habits:

Eating in the car, especially while driving

When you eat behind the wheel you are failing to concentrate on your main objective of getting to your destination safely. In addition, you become oblivious to what you eat, failing to savor the taste. You risk not even recalling the snack, only to pig out on something else later. Simply make it a rule not to allow food or eating in the car (though perhaps an exception could be made for very young passengers or passengers with low blood sugar or other conditions, who might need regular snacks during a long journey). If the driver is hungry, he or she should pull over and make a pit stop at a roadside restaurant or picnic area.

Eating while watching television

This is another example of eating while concentrating on something else and failing to process in full the activity of eating. If your favorite show is any good, you are sure to lose track of what you're putting in your mouth. If you must eat, step away from the screen. This is a terrible, widespread habit that needs to be controlled. Putting hundreds of unappreciated and possibly low-value foods and calories in your mouth just does NOT make sense in the Power of 5 lifestyle.

Bar snacks

I have been around the block and I cannot recall ever being served a healthy snack in a bar. I recommend that you bypass the bar completely. If you cannot, at least avoid the salted pretzels and Goldfish crackers.

Cocktail parties or receptions

Indulging in appetizers that don't meet the above specifications opens up a minefield of hazardous choices. Calamari might be enticing, but it is generally breaded and fried. Sometimes it is not pre-made and can be served sautéed in olive oil or with a light marinara sauce. Many people enjoy Asian cuisine, but try to keep it as clean as possible, avoiding rice and sauces.

You have a lifetime ahead of you to enjoy good health. Start making healthy choices now to discover new and healthy foods. You will find it well worth your efforts. Part 2 of this book will provide concrete recommendations toward a healthier lifestyle. It will include all you will need to get started with the Power of 5 Formula.

Power of 5 Pointers
Chapter 2- Sweets

1. *We have long known about the dangers of high fats and trans fats in our diets. Recent evidence has found sweets, sugar, high fructose corn syrup and other carbohydrates to be hazards to our health and threaten our life expectancy.*

2. *Obesity and diabetes associated with high sugar intake lead to inflammatory conditions such as coronary artery disease, cancer and neurodegenerative diseases.*

3. *Worldwide obesity rules. The rates have doubled since 1980, including in women and children in high-income countries.*

4. *A healthy lifestyle of a Mediterranean diet and increased physical activity can offset impending risks.*

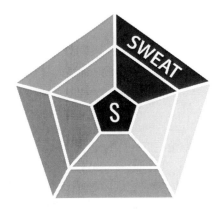

CHAPTER 3

SWEAT... Good Health Comes to Those Who Sweat

fter practicing medicine for more than thirty years, I feel I am entitled to have favorite and inspiring patients.

One such is Stanley. I took care of his brother Ron for many years as he was a long-term resident in a nursing home. Ron suffered from schizophrenia and never took care of himself. He was obese and ate uncontrollably; he developed diabetes and never exercised for a minute in the eighteen years I provided medical care to him.

Yet I was honored and delighted when Stanley became my patient well after Ron had died. While they were genetically similar as brothers, they were opposites in almost every other way. Ron had been a gifted engineer, working for a time at General Electric before he became mentally ill. Stanley has his own gifts and used them to his advantage as a New York City fireman. Stanley has always been incredibly proud of his job and the precinct in which he worked, but that does not eclipse his pride in how well he takes care of himself.

When Stanley became my patient I learned about the competitive nature of firemen and how much importance they place on the care and feeding of their most important equipment: their bodies. Stanley and the other firefighters in his department all had vigorous workout routines and kept themselves in excellent condition. They exercised four to five days a week in order to keep up with the demands of the job. Stanley would run outside in the summer and inside on a treadmill through the winter months. He ran for thirty to forty-five minutes followed by strength training for at least an hour.

The job itself put him through his paces as well. Firefighters must carry forty-five- to fifty-pound packs each time they answer a call. He and his company were responsible for the maintenance of their equipment and hoses. They would extend the heavy hoses during a fire and pull them back in afterward, often in a state of exhaustion. When Stanley retired and moved to Florida he didn't change his workout routine. He was incredibly strong, especially when it came to rowing, where he used the same muscles he had used to pull fire hoses for many years.

When Stanley became my patient he was in his late seventies. He told me he would start his day with a very healthy, high-protein breakfast, and then go to the gym. He would spend one or two hours working on all of his muscle groups. He really did not need to spend that much time at the gym, but he enjoyed exercising his jaw muscles, talking to anyone who was interested in his success story. After his workout, Stanley typically spent the day with his younger wife, who was barely able to keep up with him. He has maintained this routine well into his eighties without dropping a beat.

When I ask Stanley about his activity he tells me, "I love the way it makes me feel. I would probably have ended up like my obese, diabetic brother had I not incorporated exercising into my life. In addition, it enables me to associate with younger and vibrant people, rather than dilapidated ones my own age."

Stanley is one of many delightful examples of the importance of sweat and physical activity as part of the formula for remain youthful and AGE GRACEFULLY®.

In the past century, our society has gone through tremendous changes. Along with the development of technology to make our lives longer and better, there has been a shift from a rural farming society to a more urban manufacturing society, and then a further shift to technology and service provision. In the 1900s the average life expectancy was sixty-five years. As primarily rural dwellers, we ate mainly organic foods, worked long hours and relied on our feet to get us from place to place.

In the U.S., the development of the interstate highway system and a spike in the post-World War II production of automobiles ensured that we walked less. Consequently, our average daily energy expenditure dropped, although we ate the same diet. Over time, we walked even less and expended fewer calories while fast-food restaurants sprang up everywhere. As a result, our diets shifted, delivering more and more calories. Over the years, portion sizes also increased. During the same period, the development of cable TV and an explosion in the number of television stations presented us with more home entertainment than ever before. We became a sedentary society, we began to work longer hours, and we expended fewer calories.

Public schools shifted their focus away from physical education (and the arts), and individual fitness was neither taught nor stressed. Health classes were given very little emphasis. We became a society that watched TV and played video games. Not surprisingly, healthcare expenditures increased, with very little to show for the higher cost when compared to the health conditions in many other developed countries. And all the while, in this country the rates of obesity and chronic conditions such as cardiovascular disease and diabetes skyrocketed.

Exercise for Health

Physical activity is any bodily movement produced by skeletal muscles that results in an expenditure of energy. Physical activity is a critical component of energy balance, a term used to describe how weight, diet, and physical activity influence health, including longevity, heart health, brain health and cancer risk.

Researchers have established that regular physical activity can improve health by:

- Helping to control weight
- Maintaining healthy bones, muscles and joints
- Reducing the risk of developing high blood pressure and diabetes
- Promoting nervous system and psychological well-being

- Reducing the risk of death from heart disease
- Reducing the risk of premature death that is often associated with chronic diseases such as diabetes mellitus, hypertensive heart disease, and cancer

I will explain some of the science behind the research and outline some of the most profound health benefits to be gained from regular physical activity. In the second part of this chapter, I will share some tips for incorporating exercise into your weekly routine.

Exercise for Longevity
Leisure-time physical activity is associated with longer life expectancy, even at relatively low levels of activity and regardless of body weight. A study led by the National Cancer Institute (NCI), (63) part of the National Institutes of Health (NIH), found that people who engaged in leisure-time physical activity had life expectancy gains of as much as 4.5 years. Researchers saw benefit even in low levels of activity. For example, people who said they got half of the recommended amount of physical activity still added 1.8 years to their lives.

Steven Moore, Ph.D., of NCI's Division of Cancer Epidemiology and Genetics, and lead author of the study, indicated that "the findings highlight the important contribution that leisure-time physical activity in adulthood can make to longevity. Regular exercise extended the lives in every group that we examined in our study—normal weight, overweight, or obese."

The relationship between life expectancy and physical activity was even stronger among those with a history of cancer or heart disease when compared with people who had no history of cancer or heart disease.

What kind of exercise works best?
Aerobic exercises are the best choice for lowering blood pressure, according to the Physical Activity and Public Health: Updated Recommendation for Adults from the American College of Sports Medicine and the American Heart Association. (64) You can try brisk walking, swimming, cycling or dancing—anything that gets your heart rate up is great.

Health professionals have stated repeatedly that walking is the best overall exercise for fitness and wellbeing. It's free and available to most people, and it can easily be tailored to the seasons (perhaps some would prefer an indoor treadmill in the winter months) and individual fitness levels.

For building muscle mass, strength training that includes weights works best. Growing muscle mass is helpful for keeping weight down and metabolism primed. See more on muscle mass below.

For flexibility and joint health, practices such as tai chi, yoga and Pilates work to maintain core strength and balance without stressing joints. Aquafit or swimming lengths will have similar benefits.

If you are generally healthy, feel free to mix it up to prevent boredom— perhaps aerobics one day and yoga or Pilates the next, then a long walk outdoors later in the week.

In the second part of this book I'll make several specific suggestions for getting the most out of your workouts.

How much exercise should you try to get?

The U.S. Department of Health and Human Services 2008 Physical Activity Guidelines for Americans** recommends that adults from ages eighteen to sixty-four engage in regular aerobic physical activity for two and a half hours at moderate intensity—or one hour and fifteen minutes at vigorous intensity— each week. Moderate activities are those during which a person could talk but not sing. Vigorous activities are those during which a person could say only a few words without stopping for breath.

The large-scale study published early in 2015 by JAMA Internal Medicine, mentioned earlier, suggests that this ideal dose of exercise for a long life is a bit more than many of us currently believe we should get, but less than many of us might expect. The study also found that prolonged or intense exercise is unlikely to be harmful and could add years to people's lives. (65)

Using this data, the researchers separated the adults into three groups: those who exercised a moderate amount each week, those who did not exercise at all and those who worked out for ten times the current recommendations or more. (Meaning that they exercised moderately for a minimum of twenty-five hours per week.) They then compared fourteen years' worth of death records for the group. They found that the people who did not exercise at all were at the highest risk of early death. But those who exercised a little, not meeting the recommendations but still doing something, lowered their risk of premature death by twenty percent.

Those who met the guidelines precisely, completing 150 minutes per week of moderate exercise, enjoyed greater longevity benefits and thirty-one percent less risk of dying during the fourteen-year period compared with those who never exercised.

The sweet spot for exercise benefits, however, came among those who tripled the recommended level of exercise, working out moderately, mostly by walking for 450 minutes per week, or a little more than an hour per day. Those people were thirty-nine percent less likely to die prematurely than people who never exercised. Premature deaths are deaths that occur before a person reaches an expected age, for instance, age seventy-five. Many of these deaths are considered to be preventable. In 1900 the average life expectancy in the United States was 47 and in 1950 it was 68.2. As a result of medical technology this number has risen to 78.8 in 2015. This rise has occurred despite the adoption of sedentary lifestyles and the fast-food culture in which we live today.

The Importance of Building Muscle Mass

The more muscle older adults have, the lower their risk of death, according to a study published in the American Journal of Medicine. (66)

Researchers analyzed data from more than 3,600 older adults—ages fifty-five for men and sixty-five for women—who took part in the U.S. National Health and Nutrition Examination Survey between 1988 and 1994. The investigators used a follow-up survey done in 2004 to determine how many of the participants had died of natural causes and how muscle mass (the amount of muscle relative to height) was related to death risk. People with the highest levels of muscle mass were significantly less likely to have died than those with the lowest levels of muscle mass.

According to study co-author Dr. Arun Karlamangla, an associate professor in the geriatrics division at University of California, Los Angeles School of Medicine, "The greater your muscle mass, the lower your risk of death. Rather than worrying about weight or body mass index, we should be trying to maximize and maintain muscle mass."

Exercise for Memory, Brain Health, Mood and Creativity

For many years, scientists have linked physical exercise to brain health. In fact, compelling evidence shows that physical exercise helps build a brain that not only resists shrinkage, but also has increased cognitive abilities. We now know that exercise promotes a process known as neurogenesis, i.e. your brain's ability to adapt and grow new brain cells, regardless of your age.

John J. Ratey, a psychiatrist who wrote the book *Spark: The Revolutionary New Science of Exercise and the Brain*, revealed overwhelming evidence that exercise produces large cognitive gains and helps fight dementia. He describes research that_shows that those who exercise have a greater volume of gray matter in the hippocampal region of their brains, which is important for memory. (67)

The benefits don't stop there. Research has demonstrated that consistent aerobic exercise leads to persistent beneficial behavioral and neural plasticity in the circuits of the brain. Such exercise also produces long-term benefits that include increased neuron growth, increased neurological activity, improved stress coping and enhanced cognitive control over behavior, as well as improved declarative (facts and verbal knowledge) and working memory. (68)

People who regularly participate in aerobic exercise have greater scores on neuropsychological function and performance tests. Examples of aerobic exercise that produce these changes are running, jogging, brisk walking, swimming, and cycling. More pronounced improvements in measures of neuropsychological performance are observed in endurance athletes as compared to recreational athletes or sedentary individuals. This improvement suggests that the more exercise you get, the greater the benefits for your brain. (69)

Exercise Prevents Both Brain *and* Muscle Decay

Brain-derived neurotrophic factor, known as BDNF, is a growth factor protein that, in humans, is encoded by the BDNF gene.

Showing the interconnectedness between muscle and brain health, BDNF also expresses itself in the critical neuro-muscular system, where it protects neuro-motors from degradation. Without the neuro-motor, your muscle is like an engine without an ignition. Neuro-motor degradation is part of the process that explains age-related muscle atrophy.

BDNF is actively involved in both your muscles *and* your brain, and this cross-connection appears to be a major part of the explanation for why a physical workout can have such a beneficial impact on your brain tissue. It, quite literally, helps prevent, and even reverse, brain decay as much as it prevents and reverses age-related muscle decay. The most important message from studies like these is that **mental decline is by no means inevitable, and that exercise is as good for your brain as it is for the rest of your body.** Firefighter Stanley offers us a good example of this truth.

Exercise Helps with Stress and Depression

Exercise also has a marked, persistent, antidepressant effect in humans, an effect also believed to be facilitated through enhanced BDNF signaling in the brain. Such intracellular signaling is critical for plasticity and neuron survival.

Aerobic exercise especially is a potent long-term antidepressant and a short-term euphoriant, but any kind of consistent exercise has also been shown to produce general improvements in mood and self-esteem in all individuals. (70)

Several systematic reviews have analyzed the potential for physical exercise in the treatment of depressive disorders. The 2013 Cochrane Collaboration review of primary research on physical exercise for depression noted that, based upon limited evidence, exercise is comparable in effectiveness to psychological or antidepressant drug therapies. (71)

One of the ways exercise promotes mental health is by normalizing insulin resistance and boosting the natural "feel good" hormones and neurotransmitters associated with mood control. These include endorphins, serotonin, dopamine, glutamate, and the calming amino acid known as GABA. Exercising your muscles actually helps rid your body of stress chemicals that can lead to depression.

Other research studies have also shown clear links between inactivity and depression.

Boost Creativity—Get Moving!

Exercise can also boost your creativity, and help you come up with new solutions to problems. For example, researchers at Stanford University found that walking can increase creativity up to sixty percent. Even a casual stroll around your office can be helpful.

While the exact science behind it remains inconclusive, abundant anecdotal evidence demonstrates that exercise boosts creativity and creative thinking, regardless of the type and locale of the exercise, and that the positive effects linger for a time, even after the activity has ceased. (72)

The Impact of Exercise on Specific Health Conditions
Exercise and Hypertension

Researchers have spent decades developing new treatments for high blood pressure, but exercise is still one of the best remedies around. A single workout can reduce blood pressure for an entire day, and regular exercise can keep the pressure down over the long run.

What's more, low to moderate intensity training appears to be as beneficial— if not more so—as higher intensity training for reducing blood pressure in people with hypertension, according to the American College of Sports Medicine's guidelines on exercise and hypertension. After analyzing fifteen studies on exercise and high blood pressure, reviewers concluded that exercise training lowers blood pressure in a full seventy-five percent of people with hypertension.

Of course, exercise has many benefits beyond reducing blood pressure. Even if blood pressure doesn't budge, exercise may strengthen heart muscle, lower cholesterol, help keep weight in check, and decrease the risk of developing diabetes. The benefits extend to stroke survivors as well: Guidelines from the American Heart Association and the American College of Sports Medicine stress the importance of aerobic and strengthening exercises to improve overall health and reduce the risk of subsequent strokes.

Exercise and Diabetes

According to the National Institute of Diabetes and Digestive and Kidney Diseases, physical activity can help control diabetes and prevent diabetes problems. Physical activity helps maintain blood glucose levels within a target range. It also helps the hormone insulin action; promoting absorption of glucose into the body's cells, including muscles, for energy. The more muscle is developed, the more efficiently glucose is absorbed. If one's body doesn't make enough insulin, or if the insulin doesn't work the way it should, the body's cells don't use glucose. Blood glucose levels then get higher than desired (fasting glucose greater than 126), which meets the criteria for the diagnosis of diabetes.

People with diabetes who take insulin or certain diabetes medicines are more likely to have low blood glucose, also called hypoglycemia. If blood glucose levels drop too low, an individual can pass out, have a seizure, or go into a coma. Physical activity can make hypoglycemia more likely or worse in people who take insulin or certain diabetes medicines, so planning ahead is key.

Physical activity works together with healthy eating and diabetes medicines to prevent diabetes problems. Studies show that people with type-2 diabetes who lose weight with physical activity and make healthy changes to their eating plan are less likely to need diabetes and heart medicines. A team of healthcare professionals can help design a healthy eating plan and adjust medicines, taking into account physical activity. (73)

Exercise and Coronary Disease

As mentioned previously, routine physical activity can lower many coronary heart disease risk factors, including "bad" cholesterol, high blood pressure, and excess weight.

Aerobic exercise, such as brisk walking, is any exercise in which your heart beats faster and you use more oxygen than usual. Everyone should try to participate in moderate-intensity aerobic exercise for at least two and a half hours per week, or vigorous aerobic exercise for an hour and fifteen minutes per week. The more active you are, the more you will benefit.

The President's Council on Fitness, Sport and Nutrition (74) and the National Institute on Aging (75) both offer excellent free information and tips about the benefits of physical activity for preventing coronary and other chronic diseases.

Patients with heart conditions should consult with their physician or health team about which kinds of exercises are safe.

Here is a word or two about Herbert. After doing all his research to help his wife recover from her breast cancer, he started a much more vigorous exercise program. He started with daily workouts of just thirty minutes and within three months he was up to ninety minutes a day, five days a week. He included cardio and strength exercises, some of which will be described later in this and other chapters in this book.

Exercise and Neurodegenerative diseases—
Alzheimer's, Vascular Dementia and Parkinson's disease

After taking care of Jennie for thirty years I had become very well acquainted with her family and psychosocial history. I was aware that she had family who lived in the New York area and they had a close relationship. At some point I noted a change that bothered me. She is an athletic woman who takes great pride in in her physical appearance and is quite proud of how she looks in her late eighties. She is slender, with very little fat on her body. From the time we first met she would tell me about the exercise program she follows. While I don't remember all the details, she would go to a facility that had exercise classes including yoga, spinning, treadmill and Pilates. She would exercise in this fashion at least five days a week. She ate a very healthy diet to complement what she was doing with her exercise program. She kept her mind engaged by attending community lectures and remained very engaged with the younger women in her exercise classes.

At some point in her mid-eighties she noticed her short-term memory and cognitive functioning had changed. Over the course of the next five years I noticed this decline and even had some informants confirm this. What is interesting about the situation for Jennie is that her cognitive and mental decline has been relatively slow compared with that which any other older adults suffered.

I can't help but credit her physical activity and excellent eating habits for the slower trajectory of her mental decline.

Physical activity has been seen to improve cognitive function and has been recommended by many authorities who evaluate and treat dementias. At the 2015 Alzheimer's Association International Conference (AAIC), three new research studies were presented that supported recommendations to exercise or increase physical activity. These types of activities might play a role in both protection of an individual's brain from Alzheimer's disease and other dementias and also promote living better with the disease. The findings presented highlight the potential value of non-drug therapies for these conditions.

The Danish Dementia Research Centre (DDRC), Copenhagen, Denmark, reported results from the Danish ADEX Study (76), the first large, controlled trial of moderate- to high-intensity exercise in people living in Denmark with mild to moderate Alzheimer's.

- People who participated in the exercise program had far fewer neuropsychiatric symptoms (such as anxiety, irritability, and depression). Those in the control group had deteriorated on measures of psychiatric symptoms, while those in the intervention group improved slightly. This led to a statistically significant difference between the two groups.
- People in a subgroup of the exercise group who attended more than eighty percent of the classes and exercised vigorously (raising their heart rate to more than seventy percent of their maximal rate) had statistically significant improvements on mental speed and attention.
- In addition, people who participated in the exercise program improved in physical fitness, physical function, dual-task performance and exercise self-efficacy.

   Researchers Laura Baker, PhD, and colleagues from Wake Forest School of Medicine, Winston-Salem, N.C., reported results of a six-month randomized controlled trial of moderate-to-high intensity aerobic exercise in sixty-five sedentary adults from fifty-five to eighty-nine years old with MCI to test whether aerobic exercise might also lower tau levels in the brain. Tau protein is a substance found in the brains of patients with Alzheimer's disease.

The researchers found that:

- Participants who completed aerobic exercise (most commonly using a treadmill) saw a statistically significant reduction in tau levels in their spinal fluid. The effect was most pronounced in adults over the age of seventy.
- Aerobic exercise significantly increased blood flow in the memory and processing centers of participants' brains, with a corresponding improvement in attention, planning, and organizing abilities referred to as "executive function."

According to the author, "This study is important because it strongly suggests a potent lifestyle intervention such as aerobic exercise can impact Alzheimer's-related changes in the brain. No currently approved medication rivals these effects."

This study is one of a growing number of affirmations about the value of physical activity and brain function.

Cerebrovascular disease, also known as stroke, is the second most common cause of dementia in older adults, behind Alzheimer's. Research suggests that reducing heart health risk factors, such as high blood pressure and high cholesterol, may reduce dementia risk, and possibly even slow down the progression of cognitive decline due to mini-strokes, known as vascular cognitive impairment (VCI).

It is known that aerobic exercise decreases heart health risk factors, but it had also been thought that it would improve brain structure and function as well.

At AAIC 2015, Liu-Ambrose and colleagues reported results from a six-month study of seventy-one adults fifty-six to ninety-six years old with confirmed cases of mild VCI. (77) Participants were assigned to two groups. One did supervised aerobic exercise three times per week for sixty minutes with certified fitness instructors; the other received usual care plus an education seminar on nutrition once per month.

The researchers found that study participants who took the aerobics classes significantly improved their cognitive function, including memory and selective attention, compared with the people receiving usual care. In addition, functional brain scans acquired before and after the six-month study showed that the brains of study participants became more efficient with aerobic exercise training.

Neuroprotective Benefits of Exercise for People With Parkinson's
Exercise is an important part of healthy living for people with Parkinson's disease. Exercise is not only healthy but vital component to maintaining balance, mobility and daily living activities. Most experts believe exercise is important to good outcomes in Parkinson's, and the data supports that. Doing exercise is associated with a better sense of well-being.

There are two ways in which exercise might be helpful to Parkinson's patients:

Symptom management

Research has shown that exercise can improve gait, balance, tremor, flexibility, grip strength, and motor coordination. Exercise such as treadmill training and biking have all been shown to benefit, as have tai chi and yoga (although more studies are needed).

Possibly slowing disease progression

There is a strong consensus among physicians and physical therapists that improved mobility decreases the risk of falls and some other complications of Parkinson's. Practicing movement—physical therapy, occupational therapy, and participating in an exercise program—improves mobility. We also know that people who exercise intensely, for example by doing things like running or riding a bicycle, have fewer changes in their brains caused by aging.

Exercise

- The best way to achieve these benefits is to exercise on a consistent basis.
- Greater intensity equals greater benefits.
- Intense exercise is exercise that raises your heart rate and makes you breathe heavily. Studies have focused on running and bicycle riding, but experts feel that other intense exercise should provide the same benefit.
- More specific suggestions later in this chapter: incorporating movement and concentration to stimulate neuroplasticity and neurogenesis or what I refer to as brain-body integrative exercises.

Exercise and Cancer

Edna had been diagnosed with stage-three breast cancer. She had favorable hormone levels in the cancer tissue but still had to undergo a mastectomy and chemotherapy. Herbert did his research and found the very favorable effects of exercise on cancer recovery. I was not surprise to hear that after he presented the result of his study to Edna she found herself making major lifestyle changes that included a low-carbohydrate diet and ninety minutes of exercise five days a week.

Currently, several National Cancer Institute-funded studies are exploring the role of physical activity in cancer survivorship and quality of life, cancer risk, and the needs of populations at increased risk.

Nonetheless, there is already convincing evidence that physical activity is associated with a reduced risk of cancers of the colon and breast. Several studies have also reported links between physical activity and a reduced risk of cancers of the prostate, lung and lining of the uterus (endometrial cancer). Here's what researchers have discovered so far:

The relationship between physical activity and colon cancer risk (78)
Colorectal cancer has been one of the most extensively studied cancers in relation to physical activity, with more than fifty studies examining this association. Many studies in the United States and around the world have found that adults who increase their physical activity, either in intensity, duration or frequency, can reduce their risk of developing colon cancer by thirty to forty percent relative to those who are sedentary. This result is regardless of body mass index (BMI), with the greatest risk reduction seen among those who are most active.

The benefits appear to be greatest with high-intensity activity, although the optimal levels and duration of exercise are still hard to determine due to differences between studies, making comparisons difficult. And it is not yet clear at this time whether physical activity has a protective effect for rectal cancer, adenomas, or polyp recurrence.

Physical activity may protect against colon cancer and tumor development through its role in energy balance, hormone metabolism and insulin regulation, and by decreasing the time the colon is exposed to potential carcinogens. Physical activity has also been found to alter a number of inflammatory and immune factors, some of which may influence colon cancer risk.

The relationship between physical activity and breast cancer risk

The relationship between physical activity and breast cancer incidence has been extensively studied, in more than sixty studies published across North America, Europe, Asia, and Australia. Most studies indicate that **physically active women have a lower risk of developing breast cancer than inactive women.** However, the amount of risk reduction achieved through physical activity varies widely—between twenty and eighty percent, depending on the study. Although most evidence suggests that physical activity reduces breast cancer risk in both premenopausal and postmenopausal women, high levels of moderate and vigorous physical activity during adolescence may be especially protective. A lifetime of regular, vigorous activity is thought to be of greatest benefit; however, women who increase their physical activity after menopause may also experience a reduced risk compared with inactive women.

Existing evidence shows a decreasing risk of breast cancer as the frequency and duration of physical activity increase. Most studies suggest that thirty to sixty minutes per day of moderate- to high-intensity physical activity is associated with a reduction in breast cancer risk.

Researchers have proposed several biological mechanisms to explain the relationship between physical activity and breast cancer development. Physical activity may prevent tumor development by lowering hormone levels, particularly in premenopausal women; lowering levels of insulin, improving the immune response, and assisting with weight maintenance to avoid a high body mass and excess body fat.

The relationship between physical activity and risk of endometrial cancer

About twenty studies have examined the role of physical activity on endometrial cancer risk. The results suggest an inverse relationship between physical activity and endometrial cancer incidence. These studies suggest that women who are physically active have a twenty percent to forty percent reduced risk of endometrial cancer, with the greatest reduction in risk among those with the highest levels of physical activity.

Changes in body mass and changes in the levels and metabolism of the sex hormones such as estrogen are the major biological mechanisms thought to explain the association between physical activity and endometrial cancer.

However, the potential effect of postmenopausal hormone use, which may increase the risk of endometrial cancer, has not been fully considered in all studies.

The relationship between physical activity and lung cancer risk

At least twenty-one studies have examined the impact of physical activity on the risk of lung cancer. Overall, these studies suggest an inverse association between physical activity and lung cancer risk, with the most physically active individuals experiencing about a twenty percent reduction in risk. An analysis of many existing studies found evidence that higher levels of physical activity protect against lung cancer. But most studies have not been fully able to chart the effects of smoking or respiratory disease in estimating the magnitude of the potential benefit. In addition, the relationship between physical activity and lung cancer risk is less clear for women than it is for men.

The relationship between physical activity and risk of prostate cancer

Research findings are less consistent about the effect of physical activity on prostate cancer, with at least thirty-six studies in North America, Europe, and Asia. Overall, the research does not indicate that there is an inverse relationship between physical activity and prostate cancer. Although it is possible that men who are physically active experience a reduction in risk of prostate cancer, the potential biological mechanisms that may explain this association are unknown. They may be related to changes in hormones, energy balance, insulin-like growth factors, immunity, and antioxidant defense mechanisms. One recent study suggested that regular vigorous activity could slow the progression of prostate cancer in men age sixty-five or older.

Exercise and surviving cancer

Research indicates that physical activity after a diagnosis of breast cancer may be beneficial in improving quality of life by reducing fatigue and assisting with energy balance. One study found that women who exercised moderately (the equivalent of walking three to five hours per week at an average pace) after a diagnosis of breast cancer had improved survival rates compared with more sedentary women. The benefit was particularly pronounced in women with hormone responsive tumors.

Another study found that a home-based physical activity program had a beneficial effect on the fitness and psychological wellbeing of previously sedentary women who had completed treatment for early-stage through stage-2 breast cancer.

Increasing physical activity may influence insulin and leptin levels and thus influence breast cancer prognosis. Although there are several promising studies, it is too early to draw any strong conclusions regarding physical activity and breast cancer survival.

Two additional studies have suggested a protective association of physical activity after colon cancer diagnosis and survival. Researchers examined the relationship between levels of physical activity both before and after a diagnosis of colon cancer in two different observational studies. Whereas levels of pre-diagnosis physical activity were not related to survival, **participants with higher levels of physical activity post-diagnosis were less likely to have a cancer recurrence and enjoyed increased survival rates**.

Although these studies are promising and suggest protective effects of physical activity, more research is needed to truly understand what levels of physical activity provide these benefits.

Stay Healthy and Sharp into Old Age—Exercise!

One of the many great role models I've had in my professional life was Dr. Richard Beebe. He was chairman of the Department of Medicine at Albany Medical College for nearly thirty years and retired at the age of ninety, two years <u>after</u> he broke his hip. The stimulation and rewards of providing medical care to human beings was a vital stimulus to this man's retaining his cognitive capacity.

Two other such individuals I have known who maintained high levels of intellectual stimulation are Julie and Billy.

Julie and Billy are a delightful couple in my practice. They're both highly educated, with advanced degrees. Julie is very proud of her marine biology experience both in the lab and underwater.

Billy's experience working for NASA is quite remarkable in that he tells me he was involved in designing several components in the Apollo spacecraft. This is no small accomplishment. Both of them aged fairly well, each having their own cluster of medical problems. A few years ago Julie underwent an open-heart operation and she physically recovered as if it was the simplest appendectomy. You have to know Julie, because she has a lot to say from her perspective about how she recovered. Julie talks a lot.

I'm very patient with Julie and with Billy as sometimes they tell very long stories about very short subjects. They are lovely patients. What is so delightful about them is how they've gone about keeping their minds sharp. They work at it. They attend classes and lectures in the community. I see them at religious activities when most of the attendees are young adults or middle-aged. They, in their late eighties, show up like it's nothing. Some of these events present very complex and challenging material, yet Julie and Billy are able to process this without any trouble. When they come to office visits, they usually tell me they are reading very up-to-date books about complex people or historic events. When I question them about what they read, there is no question they are digesting the information thoroughly.

Billy has been part of the Coast Guard Auxiliary for most of his adult life. He continues to put on his uniform once a week to do his volunteer work. Julie tells me she loves to see him in uniform.

The question is how they do it. How do they maintain their cognitive function and ability to process complex information?

I can come up with several explanations. One is that they worked out. Whether it's effective or not, they do puzzles. They talk to each other about complex issues, and what I think might be the most telling is that for the last thirty years they look forward to their twice-weekly sessions of square dancing. Not only do they get the physical workout of this activity, but the cognitive challenge of remembering the steps and sequences of these dances no doubt stimulates their brain. Furthermore, this activity enables them to develop new brain pathways and utilize existing ones.

When I think about the expression "use it or lose it," I realize Billy and Julie exercise their brains so they continue to function well and stay sharp.

We certainly can all identify many individuals in our lives who retired, stopped higher- level thinking, neglected to exercise and had their brains literally and figuratively "turned to mush."

While it's never too late to start exercising, the earlier you begin and the more consistent you are, the greater your long-term rewards will be. Having an active lifestyle is really an investment in your future wellbeing, both physical and mental. I believe that, overall, high-intensity interval training really helps maximize the health benefits of exercise, while simultaneously being the most efficient, and therefore requiring the least amount of time. That said, ideally you'll want to strive for a varied and well-rounded fitness program that incorporates a wide variety of exercises.

I also strongly recommend that you avoid sitting as much as possible, and that everyone make a point of walking more every day. A fitness tracker or pedometer can be very helpful for this. I suggest aiming for 7,000 to 10,000 steps per day, *in addition to* your regular fitness regimen, not in lieu of it. Do it for your body, but also do it for your mental and cognitive health. The science is really clear on this point: you do not have to lose your mind with advancing age. Your brain has the capacity to regenerate and grow throughout the entire human lifespan, and exercise is perhaps the most potent way to ensure your brain's continued growth and rejuvenation.

A most gratifying experience for any professional, including me as a physician, is seeing the fruits of his/her labor. Observing the success that Stanley had for a lifetime of exercise and fitness has been overwhelming for me. One can read about the science supporting the concepts of the benefits of exercise but to witness it is another thing altogether and very special to me. It enables me to use this example to counsel others.

Jennie demonstrated that maintaining a diverse exercise program that includes cardiovascular, strength and flexibility activities can be extremely effective in avoiding or delaying cognitive decline. Herbert and Edna have become motivated by reality and are now about to make the serious lifestyle changes needed to combat or delay their own illnesses. When Sara, whom I will describe at the beginning of the next section revamped her life by engaging in an aggressive diet and exercise program she experienced real success. Her transformation provoke in me the type of emotions I'd feel as if I'd cured her of a serious illness.

In the next section of this chapter I will introduce my formula with remedies, along with several other patients who have made a difference by adjusting their own formulas. There will be a variety of options for staying fit and sweating. Remember, good things come to those who sweat.

S is for Sweat - Formula
The Joys of Physical Activity

Sara has been a patient for a number of years. I suspect we became acquainted through some interaction we had because she worked in a resource, in a research capacity, at the hospital in which I practiced medicine. She has dedicated her life to be a supportive wife raising two children, and working as a nurse providing research services to the hospital. In the process, she obtained a PhD.

The challenge I had with her as a patient was that she was overweight and had high blood pressure. In addition, at times her job was stressful, a situation that may have prompted her higher blood pressure. When all of her academic goals and professional accomplishments were achieved, what was lacking was attention to her health. It was as if she woke up one day and finally decided to take my advice. She proceeded to change her diet, hire a personal trainer and start to exercise. Lo and behold, it worked! She started to lose weight, become more fit and even admitted that she felt better. She told me that it took a long time for my recommendations to kick in. She needed to develop habits and wait for them to become ingrained. Once that happened, exercising became part of her lifestyle and she couldn't think of going a day, a week, a month without maintaining the fairly rigid program she and her trainer put together. Each time she came to see me as her weight decreased and she achieved her goals, her facial expression glowed with the joy of achievement.

Here's a not-so-secret tip. In order to increase your level of physical fitness, your chosen activities have to be **fun** or **enjoyable.** Otherwise, you might not bother to continue, even when you understand the tremendous health benefits you derive from getting more exercise. People who have been active all their lives have many activities to choose from. For those who have never exercised or been active, it is much harder to find activities that will enhance health or meet the exercise specifications that I outlined previously in this chapter on sweat.

When setting a goal of 150 to 450 minutes of physical activity per week, keep in mind how important it is to have enjoyable and variable choices. In addition to avoiding the boredom associated with doing the same routine every day, your body becomes accustomed to routine and develops enhanced efficiencies. You may thus burn fewer calories than if you incorporate some variability in your exercise regime.

Another important consideration when starting an exercise program is safety. If increasing physical activity and exercise is a new concept to you, I suggest booking a consultation with a physician about the safety of starting such a program. Supervision with a personal trainer or taking a class to ensure the activity is performed correctly, with proper technique, is a great idea when learning something new. Periodically, check in with the trainer again to make any necessary changes so you can maintain an effective program over time.

Personally, when I resumed outdoor bicycle riding, I visited a local cycle shop for a bicycle tune-up, but also to have my seat and handlebars adjusted in order to reduce the risk of injury. While I was there, in-store cycling experts gave me several additional pointers to enhance the benefits of riding. I was also fitted for and bought a new, more up-to-date helmet. I recalled the words of one of my good friends, who fell off his bicycle several years ago. He claims that had he not been wearing his helmet, he would have sustained a serious brain injury that could have permanently affected his life.

Another important feature for staying safe while following an exercise program is to begin each session with a proper **pre-workout routine** that includes **warming up and stretching**. This process prepares the system for activity. It increases blood supply to the extremities, gradually increases the heart rate, and gets the brain as well into a different gear.

I recall a patient of mine who found that he developed chest pressure when he started his daily walk. It lasted for only the first seven or eight minutes of his sixty-minute walk, but it concerned him. I felt the problem arose from the sudden rise from his resting heart rate to the exercise rate. He had been leaving his home without warming up and gradually increasing his heart rate. My conclusion was that when he took corrective action with a brief warm up, allowing for a gradual increase in his heart rate, his chest pressure resolved.

This warm-up period should last as long as you feel it takes to increase your heart rate and feel that you are prepared to continue.

A proper post-workout routine is just as important, perhaps even more so. Taking time to allow the heart to return to a near baseline level is important to avoid the lightheadedness or dizziness associated with blood being shunted away from the head as the muscles are exercised. During this period of time it is helpful to stretch all the muscles that have been used in the activity to reduce cramping and allow for recovery.

In an effort to balance your exercise program, try to find activities that are low impact. With the **Power of 5** formula, I provide suggestions to lead you to a healthier and longer life. However, I recognize the contradiction of recommending activities and then putting individuals at risk for ailments associated with high impact on bones and joints. There are plenty of activities to go around, so don't select only the ones that could potentially cause long-term overuse injuries. While I would not discourage running/jogging altogether, I would suggest that it not be done on hard surfaces and not be the only activity you select to promote better health.

Also consider the amount of time you devote to physical activity. As I mentioned earlier in this book, the current recommendations from major institutional bodies is 150 minutes per week. This works out to thirty minutes five days a week. With a little planning, anyone should be able to do this. But based on the more up-to-date studies I've read, 450 minutes a week or ninety minutes five days a week is the optimum goal. (79) It is clearly much harder for most of us to squeeze that amount of exercise time into our busy schedules.

Bear in mind that activity does not have to be completed all at once, nor does it have to be limited to just five days (even though rest days are also important). One suggestion would be to divide the activity into a sixty-minute endurance activity such as walking, and thirty minutes of a moderate activity such as strength training or yoga.

Types of exercise activity
Cardio and aerobic

Most people are well acquainted with cardio or aerobic exercise. There are so many to choose from: to name just a few—running/jogging, bicycling/spinning, Zumba or aerobics exercise classes, in-line skating/roller skating, swimming. To preserve the joints I usually recommend choosing the lowest impact activities possible. The idea is for the exercise to help you maintain cardiac fitness by achieving a continuous heart rate between seventy and eighty percent of maximum predicted heart rate. The easy way to calculate this is 220 minus your age = 100 percent of maximum predicted heart rate (women: same formula and multiply by .85).

Example: for a sixty-year-old man the calculation is 220 minus 60 = 160 (for a sixty-year-old woman 220 minus 60 = 160 times .85 = 136. for the man to achieve seventy-five percent of maximum heart rate he would have to get his heart rate to 120 beats a minute and for the woman it would be 102 beats a minute.

I would suggest trying to reach this level of activity for thirty to sixty minutes, five days a week to build toward your weekly total of 150 to 450 minutes.

Strength training

Another physician I know well, approximately ten years older than me, started doing bodybuilding in his mid to late forties. Although he was a man of short stature, he propped himself up and looked like a million bucks. He called his own shots with regard to the time he spent working on his physique and competing. At the time of his retirement he still looked fifteen years younger than me and could've continued to practice longer had he wished.

There is a certain grind associated with providing medical care to very sick individuals, such as he provided, and it did take its toll on him. I was proud of him because he had other outside interests, and his retirement would be one filled with both intellectual stimulation and good physical conditioning.

Strength training is any practice or exercise specifically designed to increase muscle tone, strength, and fitness. It usually includes working with weights or exercise machines or resistance tools. And research is pretty clear about the importance of it.

Since we lose one percent of our muscle mass every year, starting at age forty, we should not neglect this important activity. It is also important for maintaining bone mass.

This kind of activity does not require a gym membership, but it's very helpful to do a bit of reading in order to understand proper technique. You might want to enlist the services of an experienced personal trainer or physical therapist to provide appropriate instruction and supervision at the start of your training. Beginning with lightweight (one or two-pound) dumbbells and progressing to heavier weights is one way to start. Another option would be to use elastic resistance bands, finding a routine to work both the upper and lower body.

Flexibility training

There are several types to choose from, such as static and dynamic stretching and isometric exercises. Much like strength training, these activities do not necessarily require a gym membership and can be done in the privacy of your home. Many fine books and video programs outline the postures and routines. You can easily obtain these from libraries, from bookstores and on public and cable TV stations. Flexibility training may also be inherent in some practices such as yoga and Pilates (more on these later).

Recreational exercise

The most accessible activities can be as simple as just walking. You might include more challenging pursuits such as hiking or mountain climbing. Just choose to do something outdoors, with an abundance of fresh air and sunshine, to reap wonderful benefits. Use your imagination to come up with a long list of other potential activities you'd like to try: kayaking/canoeing, sailing, orienteering. For those with outdoor hobbies such as bird watching or photography, combining them with some type of physical activity will contribute to enhanced health and wellbeing.

Social and team activities

Here I would include many of the popular individual or team sporting activities such as bowling, golf, tennis, or ballroom dancing. Another option is that you might simply go to a nightclub to really work those legs and arms to the beat of your favorite music.

My Favorite Five

In this next section I would like to highlight five different and beneficial activities that I have personally performed and find that almost anyone can do. All of these activities can be included in the weekly goal of reaching 150 to 450 minutes of physical exercise.

They are:

1. Yoga
2. Pilates
3. Strength- Training-- Circuit or Interval Training in twenty-five-minute cycles
4. Brain-Body Integrative Exercises
5. Cycling or spinning

Yoga

I have always been very partial to yoga. This Hindu spiritual discipline utilizes breath control, simple meditation, and the adoption of specific body postures. It is widely practiced around the world for health and relaxation. Ever since one of my favorite patients reminded me that "Yoga is a non-judgmental activity. No one will ever judge you for how much or little flexibility you have," I have been comfortable participating in this type of gentle group activity. Yoga can be done in a studio setting, or at home, following a program from a book, a purchased video, or a cable TV station. YouTube has hundreds of videos as well. Be prepared to perspire, grunt and groan, but you will feel great when the session is over.

Here are some of the benefits of incorporating yoga into your activity program:

- **Improves cardiovascular health**. Hypertension is due to a constriction of blood vessels, and heart disease is due to blockage in the coronary arteries. Practicing yoga gently relaxes the blood vessels and reduces blood pressure, at the same time that it increases blood flow to the heart muscle.

- **Curbs chronic neck and low back pain**. Postures are the backbone of yoga; a regular practice is good for your stance. Besides straightening your slouch, it may also ease chronic pain. In yoga practice, when you hold a pose, your muscles contract and then slowly relax as you breath in and out. When relaxation sets in, back pain abates.

- **Sharpens the brain**. Regular yoga practice doesn't just make only your body more flexible. It does the same thing to your brain. Graham McDougall Jr., Ph.D., the lead researcher of a report published in the June 2015 issue of the *Journal of Neuroscience Nursing*, notes that participants of his yoga benefits study saw significant gains in memory performance and had fewer depressive symptoms as well. (80)

- **Controls diabetes**. A study published in the April 2015 issue of the *Journal of Clinical and Diagnostic Research* supports this finding. It describes thirty men with Type-2 diabetes who practiced yoga for six months; each saw a significant decrease in his blood glucose levels. (81)

- **Staves off stress and anxiety**. I often feel a soothing wave wash over me immediately during and after yoga practice—and it's not just a placebo effect. A new report presented at the Anxiety and Depression Association of America (ADAA) Conference 2015 linked yoga to lower levels of the stress hormone cortisol, especially in women at risk for mental health problems. (82)

- **Decreases depression**. Keeping a cool head can keep you from feeling down, too. Many studies have supported this over the years. When you exercise, your body releases chemicals called endorphins. These endorphins interact with the receptors in your brain that reduce your perception of pain, and trigger a positive feeling in the body. It's the so-called "natural high" and a good way to keep anxiety and depression at bay.

- **Lowers cancer risk**. Regular yoga practice has been shown to suppress the genetic mutation that can lead to cancer. Patients may also use yoga as a fierce weapon to battle the effects of the disease and its treatment. A study published in January 2016 in *Journal of Clinical Oncology* found that women performing yoga twice a week for as little as three months lowered inflammation, boosted energy, and lifted moods. (83)

- **Promotes positive self-perception**. The word yoga itself means union. It aims to unite your mind, body and spirit. During yoga practice, we inhale positive emotions and exhale negative emotions. Yoga may also help quiet the endless to-do lists and negative self-talk of mind chatter.

Pilates

I think the general public is unaware of the physical demands on the life of a physician. As hard as physicians work, sometimes I think the public thinks they have it easy. Don't they play golf on Wednesdays, Saturdays and Sundays? I don't think they are aware of the sleep deprivation, long hours and diminished opportunities to attend exercise classes.

One of my colleagues has worked in the community for over thirty years. He has maintained a very successful practice, one which included morning hospital rounds and a full work schedule throughout the day, followed by attendance at appropriate meetings in the evening. He tried never to miss his children's athletic events or school functions, and occasionally found time to enjoy weekends with friends and family.

Although he had always been very athletic, he found he was not able to keep up with those kinds of activities during his professional career. He did attempt to eat well to maintain his weight and from time to time was able to exercise at his gym. Every now and again he'd suffer some body aches and pains and a little muscle stiffness, but these improved with rest and gentle stretching.

When he had to adapt to the use of electronic medical records and computers, monitors and keyboards, my colleague started to suffer from multiple body aches and pains and, overall, deconditioned muscles. He evaluated his workspace very carefully and even had an expert in ergonomics adjust the height of his monitor. He purchased an expensive shelf for his keyboard, attempting to reduce his back strain, to no avail. My colleague visited his orthopedist and spent a great deal of time in his physical therapist's facility. He worked on flexibility and strengthening his muscles with electronic stimulation and massages, but nothing seemed to relieve the tightness in his upper and lower back.

When we spoke I encouraged him to consider some other options. I recommended both yoga and Pilates. Introducing yoga and especially Pilates has been instrumental in changing his conditioning, improving his endurance and flexibility. These physical improvements enabled the potential to prolong his career. It certainly improved his outlook on patient care. A year and a half after starting his Pilates, he admitted he feels more productive than he had been since starting to use computers in his practice.

Over the past year, I have been having some discomfort in the area between my shoulder blades. I discovered it is at least partially an occupational hazard of being a doctor.

As a primary care physician during much of my career, I have been physically active in many ways: getting in and out of my car to visit patients in hospitals and nursing homes, running around my office all day long. Unfortunately, too much time has been spent sitting on a stool in an exam room listening to patients and preparing their charts (in the past), or using a keyboard to type my electronic medical record (the current method). It has taken a toll on my upper back and the muscles between my shoulders. Consulting with many different therapists and exercise specialists determined that Pilates has something to offer with regard to building strength and flexibility in my upper back.

Pilates is a form of exercise developed in the early 20th century by German fitness specialist Joseph Pilates. Originally designed to help rehabilitate war veterans, his system emphasizes **the balanced development of the body through core strength, flexibility, and awareness in order to support efficient, graceful movement.** The Pilates method has become one of the most popular exercise systems in the country. One of the best things about it is that it works well for a wide range of people. It has been embraced by athletes and dancers as well as seniors, women rebounding from pregnancy, and people at various stages of physical rehabilitation.

By incorporating Pilates into an exercise routine, participants get an excellent workout and a stronger core. This is important, as the core muscles in the middle of the body support the entire infrastructure of the body. In addition to better sleep and better sex, including Pilates in an activity program can deliver even more benefits:

It is a whole-body fitness program. Unlike some forms of exercise, Pilates does not over-develop some parts of the body and neglect others. While Pilates training focuses on core strength, it trains the body as an integrated whole. Pilates workouts promote strength and balanced muscle development as well as flexibility and increased range of motion for the joints.

It is adaptable to many fitness levels and needs. The foundational ideas behind Pilates movements can be applied to a senior just starting to exercise, an elite athlete or anyone in between. Building core strength, focusing on the proper alignment of the body's framework, and a body/mind integrative approach make Pilates accessible to all. Pilates workouts can be done with or without simple aids (mat class) or using sophisticated equipment such as The Reformer. But any workout can be tailored to individual needs.

It creates strength without bulk. It works toward building toned muscles that work perfectly within the context of the body as a whole, and the functional needs of individuals as they move through life. One of the ways Pilates creates long, strong muscles is by taking advantage of a type of lengthening muscle contraction called an eccentric contraction.

Pilates increases flexibility. An increase in the length and stretchiness of the muscles and a wider range of motion within the joints support a body that can stretch and bend to meet the flow of life.

Pilates develops core strength. The core muscles of the body are the deep muscles of the back, abdomen, and pelvic floor. We rely on them to support a strong, supple back, good posture, and efficient movement patterns. When the core is strong, the frame of the body is supported. This means the neck and shoulders can relax, and the rest of the muscles and joints are freed to do their jobs—and not more.

It can improve posture. Starting with movement fundamentals and through mat and equipment exercises, Pilates trains the body to express itself with strength and harmony. You can see it in the beautiful posture of those who practice Pilates.

It increases awareness and body/mind connection. Joseph Pilates was adamant that Pilates was about "the complete coordination of body, mind, and spirit." The Pilates principles he designed—for centering, concentration, control, precision, breath, and flow—are key concepts that we use to integrate body and mind.

Strength-Circuit and Interval Training

> Amanda and Manny are typical forty-year-old adults. They have been engrossed in the tasks of raising three children. Each has employment that requires a lot of responsibility. Neither of them took particularly good care of themselves, never finding the time to exercise or eat right. Arlene worked for an internal medicine physician who preached to his patients about developing healthy habits. Nothing seemed to rub off on her. Manny had poor role models pertaining to taking care of himself. In addition, he suffered with high triglycerides and never seemed to be able to restrict his diet.
>
> One day both Amanda and Manny had an epiphany of sorts and joined a gym. It was a boot camp type program with interval training. In a short time, their muscles hurt but they stuck with it. Gradual and then impressive changes took place in their physical appearance. Both indicated they developed a feeling of well-being, improved energy levels, and better overall satisfaction with their lives together. It appeared they were able to manage family matters better and found more time to spend with their children despite the added time they had spent working out in the gym. They both realized that their bodies would be even better if they also changed their dietary habits.
>
> Making appropriate changes helped them accomplish their goals. The effects of circuit training for them was dramatic. They became a team and enjoyed their additional time together.

Circuit training consists of sequentially performing multiple exercises on specific body parts with little rest in between exertions. The exercises can be performed with free-weights (two- or three-pound hand-weights, for example), or using machines designed to increase resistance and target specific muscle groups. A "circuit" is a single set of these exercises. Sets are repeated several times within a twenty-five-minute or longer period.

Interval training is a slightly different type of physical program that involves a series of low- to high-intensity exercise workouts interspersed with rest or relief periods. The high-intensity periods are typically at or close to anaerobic exercise (which means short-lasting, high-intensity activity, where the body's demand for oxygen exceeds the oxygen supply available), while the recovery periods involve activity of lower intensity. Varying the intensity of effort exercises the heart muscle, providing a cardiovascular workout, and permitting the person to exercise for longer or more intense periods of time.

Interval training can refer to the organization of any cardiovascular workout (e.g., cycling, running, rowing, etc.), and is prominent in training routines for many sports. It is a technique particularly employed by runners, but athletes in many disciplines use this type of training. Personal trainers frequently use this type of training because it affords the opportunity to vigorously exercise many different muscle groups. Most practitioners also find it helpful to have a coach standing by to administer tough love and encouragement.

Exercise caution. For circuit training to be effective, it is particularly important to establish good technique. Initially working with a trainer or instructor is a good idea. It is also important to resist the urge to rest after completing a set; maximum benefits accrue from sustaining an elevated heart rate and keeping muscles warm and primed.

Caution should also be exercised when undertaking a program of interval training in order to avoid over-exertion. Anyone with underlying health concerns should be very careful. I encourage participants to consult a physician before diving in. That advice goes for any exercise program that involves cardiovascular or high-impact activity.

The inclusion of circuit or interval training in an exercise regime squashes some of the common excuses that people use for not exercising. That's because it can take up little time, it's action packed, it does not need to be done every day, and the order, type, and intensity of exercise can be personalized.

Due to the lack of rest that circuit and interval training demands, an elevated heart rate is maintained for the entire period of exercise. This burns calories and, over time, builds cardiovascular capacity and stamina.

As a geriatrician I have reviewed the topic with regard to my older patients. It is well established that senior men and women lose one percent of muscle mass each year starting at age forty. The question that arises is whether exercise can overcome this loss of muscle mass. Several studies have concluded they can, including one in which I participated as a principal investigator many years ago. Another study performed more recently in the Department of Physical Therapy at the University of Alabama at Birmingham concluded that older adults require a higher dose of weekly loading than the young to maintain muscle mass during a progressive resistance (strength) training program, yet gains in strength among adults were well preserved and remained at or above levels of untrained young.(84)

Brain-Body Integrative Exercises

Neuroplasticity is the brain's ability to reorganize itself by forming new neural connections throughout life. It's a relatively new field of scientific investigation but it is becoming clear that forming new neural connections is a key aspect to ensuring the brain continues to develop in a favorable way as we age. Computer programs such as Lumosity (an online subscription program of cognitive games) have been developed for just this purpose.

What has also been discovered is that combining physical activity with required brain integration has been shown to promote neurogenesis (the growth and development of nervous tissue) and neuroplasticity as well. Unfortunately, the concept is not well promoted, so it's hard to find exercises that do this.

I recently discovered the book and online program, Super Body Super Brain, developed by internationally renowned personal trainer Michael Gonzalez-Wallace. (85) I found it an especially useful source of exercises that promote better brain function. The exercises in this book demand balance and concentration and not only tone the body, but increase brain activity through stimulation.

The targeted exercise circuits as described in the book can yield some of the following amazing physical benefits:

- Improved alertness and less fatigue
- Improved memory capability
- Improved mood
- Weight loss and a reduction in body fat
- Stronger core muscles
- Increased heart and lung endurance
- Improved balance and coordination
- Better posture and flexibility

Cycling or spinning

I have a patient named George and a friend named Nick. Each in his own way has taken to the sport of cycling and improved his feeling of wellbeing and self-esteem.

George is a businessman who has achieved great success during the twenty years I have been taking care of him. He travels a great deal, but when he is home he makes an appointment to avidly ride his bicycle. His weekend rides with a number of his friends and his cycling club often cover sixty miles each day at very high speeds. He enjoys the high intensity training that occurs as a result of this. He participated in several races that required meticulous attention to his diet, his speed and rest. He uses computers to calculate minor nuances that would make him more successful. He consumes so much energy in this process that at times he even had difficulty maintaining an ideal body weight. There was clearly a release of endorphins in this process, as he would describe himself as addicted to cycling. When I asked him he told me, "Riding helps keep a certain balance in my life and there is no doubt that it has helped me become more successful in other areas of my life, especially my business."

My friend Nick, with whom I play golf periodically, has included cycling as part of his exercise routine. Nick is unique among my friends because he likes to participate in triathlons. It is fairly common for me to play golf on a Saturday afternoon with Nick *after* he has ridden his bicycle for fifty or sixty miles. There is no weariness to his stride and sometimes I needle him when I tell him that during my spinning class I cycled twenty-three miles. I have watched Nick become laser focused in both his golf game and his competitiveness in triathlons. I've noticed that it has made him more energetic and more focused on his business, enabling him to have greater success. He is much more attentive to his family matters, as result of maximizing his time with them.

Cycling is essentially riding a bicycle and spinning is an indoor version that involves working out on a specialized, adapted stationary bike. Getting an endorphin rush from these types of workouts has huge side benefits. Most notably, these are very low impact activities with minimal risk for joint injury or pain. When cycling outdoors, the rider absolutely needs a well-tuned bike and headgear/helmet, but indoors, all you really need is a good attitude, a towel and a bottle of your favorite liquid to maintain hydration. In a spinning class, the leader or instructor provides music and calls out instructions to motivate riders to achieve their best workout possible. In this kind of setting it is possible to make precise adjustments to resistance and incline for a different kind of workout, and closely monitor "sprints" and warm-up/cooling down periods.

Additional benefits of cycling and spinning include:

Burned calories: A spinning class can burn on average 500 calories per session. Spinning or cycling regularly is sure to lead to a more toned physique and the replacement of excess fat with muscle.

Improved cardiovascular and respiratory health: Spinning can be performed as an anaerobic exercise, pulling energy from reserves and building up muscular endurance over an extended period of time. However, there are also aerobic benefits. Spinning classes include both endurance and cardiovascular training. Cycling can be tailored to be leisurely and social or deployed as a cardiovascular workout by using inclines in the natural landscape and modulating speed and resistance afforded by the bicycle's gear system.

Improved mood and less anxiety: The warm-up and cool down are great ways to relax. Before and after putting your body through a strenuous spinning class you can close your eyes, work just a little, and allow the physical exertion to become a catharsis for releasing pent-up emotions. Spinning also builds mental strength. The important thing is that you carry through with your regular spinning routine. Push through difficult times, work up the hill climbs and ride through the endurance training. Self-discipline of the mind gained from spinning can be applied to all areas of life. It is most beneficial in areas of self-control and confidence. Spinning really does help to develop a positive, "can do" attitude.

A great abdominal workout: In addition to the major leg muscles worked during a spinning class, the abdominal muscles also get a workout. As you ride, unlike racing a bike on the road, you get an upper body rhythm going that helps you keep your leg rhythm. The movement from a slightly bent position and side to side works both the central abdominal muscles and those along the sides of your abdomen. You may not see immediate results of your abdominal work, but over time you will feel your entire body begin to tone up, including your abdominal area.

Fun Riding Together

Regardless of fitness level, each individual works equally as hard at his or her own level. It is amazing how you can feed off the energy of other riders when you begin to fatigue and start thinking you might want to quit. Spinning alone does not offer this same effect and one is likely to quit earlier than if in a class. Riding together also gives you the opportunity to encourage others. You can inspire those who have not yet reached your level of fitness, while those stronger than you inspire you. Working together, everyone who rides can reach his or her goals.

When my colleague threw his next party, guess who sat down with my wife and me? If you guessed Herbert and Edna, you are correct. It had been five years since the previous party and three years since each had their incursion into the medical arena.

Herbert has continued to exercise five days a week, but he also instituted major changes to his diet. He eats a very low-carbohydrate, low-calorie diet; Mediterranean type foods; copious amounts of fish, some chicken and even red meat. He tells me how great he feels. Since he knew I would be in attendance, he brought me his most recent lab test. There was a complete turnaround in his cholesterol, triglycerides and even his blood sugar. His metabolic syndrome resolved with his lifestyle change. He is a remarkable success story.

Edna has had similar success. She eats most of what Herbert does, but no red meat. She exercises five days a week and has lost enough weight that she is no longer in the obese category. Her tumor markers for her breast cancer are in a range that is considered non recurrence. Both she and Herbert report that they have never been more energetic or slept as well as they do now. They are a fantastic success story.

I want to mention one additional component that they have going for them—their partnership and companionship—because I am not certain either one could have done it without the motivation they provided each other to change and extend their lives.

I will have more to say about the value of companionship in chapter six.

The information presented in this chapter demands your attention as sweat and exercise provide a cornerstone of the **Power of 5 Formula**. Remember, exercise may be the best medicine ever created.

Power of 5 Pointers
Chapter 3-Sweat

1. As a result of the development of improved transportation, our average daily energy expenditure dropped although we ate the same diet. We walked less and expended fewer calories, and fast-food restaurants sprang up everywhere. During the same period, with the development of cable TV and an explosion in the number of television stations and home computers, we became even an even more sedentary society. We now work longer hours, and we expended fewer calories.
2. Impressive scientific and epidemiologic research about the value of exercise of any type reduces one's risk of developing a chronic disease.
3. Exercises reduce the risk level for diabetes mellitus, coronary artery disease, and hypertension. In addition, exercise improves survival in cancer patients.
4. To reduce your risk set a goal of 150 to 450 minutes each week.
5. There are countless options to choose from when it comes to exercise. Find the ones you will enjoy and can do for the rest of your life.

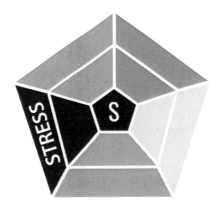

CHAPTER 4

STRESS... It Is as Bad for You as Smoking or Obesity

Barbara became a patient when she came to see me in 2001 with a case of diarrhea. She had been hospitalized in Missouri a few weeks earlier for pneumonia and had been treated with antibiotics. Diagnostic testing revealed that she also had C. difficile colitis, which required a different set of antibiotics to be taken over a prolonged period of time.

As a physician, I get to know patients pretty well when they have a prolonged hospitalization and care plan. I discovered that Barbara had contended with a great deal of stress in her life. Her brother had recently died in Missouri and left an enormous set of problems for her as executor of his estate. There were three homes and all had mortgages and were worth less than what was owed on the mortgages. It was a mess that would stress Barbara for years.

Things had not yet settled down for her when her mother became ill; she died after a long illness. Barbara confided in me that her stress was unbearable. She started to have difficulties sleeping and later suffered anxiety attacks. The stress drained her emotionally; she had difficulty controlling her appetite and had no energy for exercise, or even to complete her daily chores.

If these circumstances weren't bad enough, Barbara developed breast cancer.

I have to wonder about the impact of years of stress on her immune system, possibly leading to the development of her cancer.

As I grew up I experienced very little stress in my life. I was well aware of the stresses and hardship my parents experienced in their lives and knew how fortunate I was to have escaped the kinds of events that challenged them. I did allow myself to be in situations that provoked certain stresses, but they were generally under very controlled situations. I would think that playing high school varsity basketball was stressful, but I understood it was only a game. I would delight in the thought that I would be called upon in a critical situation to sink a winning basket. I believed that it and other situations would better prepare me for the rigors of life.

The application process for college and medical school would turn out to be a stressful one for me. Without a doubt, both the educational path leading to a medical career and the practice of medicine have their share of stress, and I feel as though I have dealt with them effectively.

When I was a medical resident I was asked to research and present information to my fellow students about stress and its impact on medical conditions. At the time, I focused on hyperventilation and the effect it had on patients' symptoms. I discovered that reports about stress and its symptoms went back millennia. I vividly recall the term, "soldier's heart," used to describe chest symptoms reported by soldiers fighting during the Civil War. Documents reveal that these soldiers were taken off the battlefield and hospitalized for extended periods of time. Most likely, these were the symptoms of stress and hyperventilation. The response to stress by breathing rapidly and expelling too much carbon dioxide caused constriction of blood vessels supplying the heart and brain, resulting in lightheadedness or a tightening feeling in the chest—much like symptoms of suffering a heart attack. Reading about soldier's heart led me to Herbert Benson's book *The Relaxation Response*, (86) which I will revisit in the second half of this chapter. Gaining an understanding about this condition was very helpful to me.

How Stress Affects the Body

The American Medical Association has noted that stress is the basic cause of more than sixty percent of all human illness and disease. Both directly and indirectly, stress has a profound impact on health and wellbeing, and we are only beginning to fully understand how this works. (87) Living GRACEfully requires us to examine this phenomenon more closely and devise strategies to offset the negative impacts of stress on the quality of an aging life.

The Science of Stress

Biological stress begins with the very basic processes in the body that produce and use energy. We eat foods and we breathe, and our body use those two vital elements (glucose from food and oxygen from the air) to produce energy in a process known as metabolism. You may already think of the word metabolism as it pertains to eating—"My metabolism is fast, so I can eat dessert," or "My metabolism has slowed down over the years, so I'm gaining weight." But since metabolism is all about energy, it also encompasses breathing, circulating blood, eliminating waste, controlling body temperature, contracting muscles, operating the brain and nerves, and just about every other activity associated with living.

These everyday metabolic activities that sustain life also create "metabolic stress," which, over time, results in damage to our bodies. Take breathing, for example. Obviously, we could not survive without oxygen, but oxygen is a catalyst for much of the damage associated with aging because of the way it is metabolized inside our cells. Tiny parts of the cell, called mitochondria, use oxygen to convert food into energy. While mitochondria are extremely efficient in doing this, they produce potentially harmful by-products called **oxygen free radicals**. A variety of environmental factors, including tobacco smoke and sun exposure, can also produce oxygen free radicals. They react with and create instability in the surrounding molecules in a process called oxidation.

Some free radicals are beneficial. The immune system, for instance, uses oxygen free radicals to destroy bacteria and other harmful organisms. Oxidation and its by-products also help nerve cells in the brain to communicate. But, in general, the outcome of free radicals is damage to other molecules, including proteins and DNA. Because mitochondria metabolize oxygen, they are particularly prone to free radical damage. As damage mounts, mitochondria may become less efficient, progressively generating less energy and more free radicals.

Scientists study whether the accumulation of oxidative damage in our cells and tissues over time might be responsible for many of the changes we associate with aging. Free radicals are already implicated in many disorders linked with advancing age, including cancer, atherosclerosis, cataracts, and neuro-degeneration.

In the early 1960s, scientists discovered that fruit flies exposed to a burst of heat produced proteins that helped their cells survive the temperature change. Over the years, scientists have found these "**heat shock proteins**" in virtually every living organism, including plants, bacteria, worms, mice, even humans. Scientists have learned that, despite their name, heat shock proteins are produced when cells are exposed to a variety of stresses, not just heat. The proteins can be triggered by oxidative stress and by exposure to toxic substances—for example, chemicals. When heat shock proteins are produced, they help cells dismantle and dispose of damaged proteins and help other proteins keep their structure and not become unraveled by stress.

Heat shock response to stress changes with age. Older animals have a higher everyday level of heat shock proteins, indicating that their bodies are under more biological stress than younger animals. On the other hand, many older animals are unable to produce an adequate amount of heat shock proteins to cope with fleeting bouts of stress from the environment.

Although considered a possible aging biomarker in animal models—something that could predict lifespan or development of age-related problems—the exact role heat shock proteins play in the human aging process is not yet fully clear.

The Stress Hormones

Thanks to the work of our sympathetic nervous system, the so-called "fight or flight" system that takes over when we're stressed, stressful triggers—both emotional and physical—can cause your body to react as if a lion is chasing you. That's due to a number of hormones that are in charge of adding fuel to the fire.

Adrenaline is a hormone produced by the adrenal glands after they receive a message from the brain that a stressful situation has presented itself. Along with norepinephrine, adrenaline is largely responsible for the immediate reactions we feel when stressed.

Imagine you're trying to change lanes in your car. Suddenly, from your blind spot, comes a car racing at 100 miles per hour. You return to your original lane and your heart is pounding, your muscles are tense, you're breathing faster, and you may be sweating. Along with the increase in heart rate, adrenaline also gives you the surge of energy you might need to run away from a dangerous situation. It also focuses your attention.

A hormone similar to adrenaline called **norepinephrine** is released from the adrenal glands and also from the brain. Its primary role is arousal. It also helps to shift blood flow away from areas where it might not be so crucial, like the skin, and toward more essential areas at the time, like muscles, so you can flee the stressful scene. Although norepinephrine might seem redundant given adrenaline (which is also sometimes called epinephrine), it is likely that we have both hormones as a type of backup system.

Cortisol is a steroid hormone also produced by the adrenal glands. It takes a little more time for the effects of cortisol to kick in because the release of this hormone requires a multi-step process involving two additional minor hormones. First, the part of the brain called the amygdala has to recognize a threat. It then sends a message to the hypothalamus, which releases corticotropin-releasing hormone (CRH). CRH then tells the pituitary gland to release adrenocorticotropic hormone (ACTH), which tells the adrenal glands to produce cortisol.

In survival mode, optimal amounts of cortisol can be lifesaving. It helps to maintain fluid balance and blood pressure, while regulating some body functions that aren't crucial in the moment, such as reproductive drive, immunity, digestion and growth.

But when you worry about something, the body continuously releases cortisol, and chronic elevated levels can lead to some serious health issues. Too much cortisol can suppress the immune system, increase blood pressure and sugar, decrease libido, produce acne and contribute to obesity.

Estrogen and testosterone are also hormones that affect how we react to stress, as are the neurotransmitters dopamine and serotonin. But the classic fight-or-flight reaction is mostly triggered by the three major players mentioned above.

Stress, Aging and Telomeres

All the cells in our body contain tiny clocks called telomeres that determine how long they will live. Telomeres are little caps at the end of chromosomes that prevent loss or injury to genetic information during cell division. Each time a cell divides, part of the telomere is lost and it becomes shorter. When a telomere eventually disappears because of repeated cell divisions, chromosomal damage prevents the cell from accurately reproducing itself. This shortening and eventual erosion of telomeres is prevented or reduced by telomerase, an enzyme in cells that preserves their length. Some research suggests that telomere destruction and reconstruction is related to the balance between aging and cancer. This could, at least partially, explain why cancer is more common in the elderly.

Short telomeres have been linked to a wide range of other human diseases, including coronary heart disease, osteoporosis and HIV infection. University of California Los Angeles researchers recently confirmed prior reports that people subjected to chronic stress tend to have shorter telomeres. They have now uncovered a mechanism that explains how stress causes telomere shortening. This could one day lead to breaking the well-known links between stress and heart disease, as well as accelerated aging. (88) (89)(90)

This study also shows that cortisol suppresses telomerase activation in immune system cells so that telomeres are no longer protected during cell division and become progressively shorter. This leads to early cell aging and distorted replicas of the original cell that could lead to cancer and other diseases. This and other studies suggest that one day a pill could be used to strengthen the immune system's ability to weather chronic emotional stress. (91) (92)

Stress and Aging

The first organism to be genetically manipulated to have a longer lifespan was a type of worm that proved to be resistant to stress caused by heat. Researchers have learned that a common thread among all long-lived animals is that their cells (and in some cases the animals as a whole) are more resistant to a variety of stresses, compared with animals that have an average or shorter lifespan. (93)

Scientists also found that age-related damage to DNA and proteins is often reversible and does not cause problems until the damage evokes a stress response. This suggests that it is the stress response, rather than the damage itself, that is partially responsible for age-related deterioration. (94)

In addition, researchers are studying the relationship between psychological stress and aging. In one study, mothers of severely and chronically sick children had shorter telomeres, relative to other women. In other research, caregivers of people with Alzheimer's disease were found to have shortened telomeres. These findings could suggest that emotional or psychological stress might affect the aging process. More research on the mechanisms involved is needed before scientists can make any conclusions about clinical implications. (95)

Stress comes in two basic flavors, physical and emotional, and both can be especially taxing for older people. As described above, the impacts of physical stress are clear. As people get older, wounds heal more slowly and colds become harder to shake. A seventy-five-year-old heart can be slow to respond to the demands of exercise. And when an eighty-year-old woman walks into a chilly room, she will need an extra-long time for her body temperature to adjust. It's no joke that our grandmothers always kept sweaters handy.

Similarly, chronic emotional stress can release lingering amounts of harmful hormones. Over time, the brain can slowly lose its skills at regulating hormone levels. As a result, older people who feel worried or anxious tend to produce larger amounts of stress hormones, and the alarm doesn't shut down as quickly as it might in someone younger. According to a study published in the journal *Psycho-neuroendocrinology*, women are especially susceptible to an overload of stress hormones as they age. The study found that the impact of age on cortisol levels is nearly three times stronger for women than for men. And when researchers checked both the telomeres and the stress levels of fifty-eight healthy premenopausal women, the stunning results revealed that, on average, the immune system cells of highly stressed women had aged by an extra ten years. (96)

That's not all. According to a recent report from the University of California at San Francisco, extra cortisol over the years can damage the hippocampus, a part of the brain that's crucial for storing and retrieving memories. (97) Several studies have found that high cortisol goes hand in hand with poor memory, so we might be able to chalk up certain "senior moments" to stress. (98)

Years of emotional distress may even increase the risk of Alzheimer's disease. A five-year study of nearly 800 priests and nuns published in the American Journal *Neurology* highlighted this potential hazard. The subjects who reported the most stress were twice as likely as the least-stressed subjects to develop the disease. (99)

Stress and Medical Illness

An essential understanding of stress is important because of its frequent occurrence and association with a variety of illnesses. These include but are not limited to cancer, cardiac disease, and a variety of autoimmune diseases. Some studies have concluded that nearly seventy-five percent of all doctor visits are stress related, and the number of people who say that they experience prolonged or frequent stress is in the hundreds of millions. **Stress is a serious health issue that impacts an enormous number of people.**

Though stress affects people on both physical and psychological levels, it can vary widely in individuals based on gender, genetics, and tolerance levels. Many people who suffer from stress can also become victims of the bad behavior often associated with stress—smoking, making poor dietary choices, and getting less than the optimal amount of sleep. All of these factors are contributors to an overall frequency and severity of many types of illnesses.

It is now clear that stress responses sent to the brain can have a dramatic negative impact on immune cells. The consequent prolonged pumping out of stress hormones can lead to autoimmune disease among people with high stress levels. Stress has been proven to both rapidly accelerate the progression of HIV/AIDS onset, and contribute to a large variety of other infections, including basic colds and flu, and some cancers that are suspected of being viral in origin, such as Kaposi's sarcoma and some lymphomas. (100)

Recent evidence also points to a broader cancer link. It is now believed that the neuroendocrine response—the release of hormones into the blood—can impair physiological processes that naturally occur to help us ward off cancers. Specifically, it is believed that this neuroendocrine responses leave our bodies weakened and can alter some of the DNA codes responsible for cell repair and regulation of physiology within the body. This means that increased stress can lead to an increased susceptibility to cancer. Furthermore, if you have cancer accompanied by chronic stress, the progression of the disease can be much faster and more severe than it would be in someone with a decreased stress level.

Stress can also contribute to cardiovascular disease. People who suffer from prolonged or excessive stress put an increased strain on the heart. Additionally, the stress response induces the secretion of glucocorticoids like glucagon and cortisone. In patients with chronically high blood pressure (often a byproduct of stress) these blood glucose molecules bind with proteins in the bloodstream. The byproduct of this process is inflammation and atherosclerosis, both serious contributing factors in cardiovascular disease.

Stress, Chronic Obstructive Pulmonary Disease (COPD) and Depression

COPD is an umbrella term used to describe progressive lung diseases including emphysema, chronic bronchitis, refractory (non-reversible) asthma, and some forms of bronchiectasis. This disease is characterized by increasing breathlessness. COPD affects 11.4 million people in the U.S. Many of these patients also suffer from anxiety and depression. A recent review of the literature confirmed that they have a higher prevalence of anxiety and depression than the general population, some of whom have other chronic diseases. It also revealed that stressed-out patients had significantly higher death rates. In another study, research demonstrated that depressive symptoms were associated with higher death rates in 121 patients with stable COPD. All were evaluated for depression, and, sure enough, approximately twenty percent were classified as having moderate to severe depression. Over the eight-and-a-half year follow-up period, seventy-six participants died, and those with clinically significant depression were found to be twice as likely to be at increased risk for death from all causes. (101)

This significant association between depression and death could not be explained by age, gender, or the severity of COPD. One explanation might be that depression disrupts hypothalamic-pituitary-adrenal activities that regulate responses to stress and immune system resistance to disease. It is well established that depression is associated with impaired immune defenses due to chronic elevated levels of cortisol. These also cause loss of memory, another common complaint in depression, which could be a factor in patients who forget to take their medications or neglect to follow medical advice. There is no good evidence that antidepressant drugs lessen these complications of depression, and many have adverse side effects that further diminish the quality of life. Furthermore, depressed patients may be less likely to take medications as prescribed, or follow other medical advice such as engaging in regular exercise or limiting smoking and drinking alcohol.

It has been noted that primary care clinicians, and especially pulmonary specialists, often report that they do not feel comfortable diagnosing or treating anxiety and depression, as this is not always part of their training. But because COPD death rates have doubled over the past thirty years, healthcare professionals need to be more aware of the connection between stress and mortality in these patients. Researchers who have worked on these studies linking COPD with depression and stress advise that patients should be screened for anxiety and depression. Those at increased risk should be referred to appropriate mental health specialists or offered other resources for further assessment and appropriate treatment.

Stress and Memory

It has been well established that stress destroys cells in the hippocampus, the brain site responsible for memory storage and retrieval. This happens to most of us as we get older, especially memory for recent events. A recent study that followed for twelve years over 1,200 senior citizens without such problems found that those who began to exhibit mild cognitive impairment due to stress or depression were much more likely to develop Alzheimer's disease. But there is also recent strong evidence that memory loss linked to increased stress is starting to surface in individuals in their forties. (102)

Though stress can be a complex contributor to a multitude of diseases, it is also something that can be managed with appropriate healthcare and effective preventative techniques. By decreasing levels of stress it is possible to decrease the risk of developing disease, and, just as importantly, decrease the odds of succumbing to the poor lifestyle choices that also contribute to disease.

In the second part of this book, I will outline some specific strategies for coping with too much stress. Diet, exercise and a positive outlook can go far to limit the damage caused by the effects of stress on the aging, as well as on loved ones and caregivers.

Emotional and Social Support

At any age, stress is a part of life. Young and old alike have to face difficult situations and overcome obstacles. Older people may face failing health or dwindling finances—or simply the challenges of retaining their independence. Unfortunately, the body's natural defenses against stress break down with age. I've noticed that seniors who manage to AGE GRACEFULLY® have a few things in common. One is that they stay connected to friends and family.

A wealth of epidemiologic data on death rates in married, single and divorced individuals as well as an abundance of psycho-physiologic and laboratory testing confirm that strong social and emotional support is a powerful factor for improving the quality of life.

Emotional support can be derived from family and friends by belonging to religious or other kinds of social communities, by being active in sports, leisure, or civic activities. Caring for someone can provide mutual emotional support; even tending to pets or plants may provide benefits.

Social support buffers the adverse effects of stress on cardiovascular and immune responses, and can provide numerous health benefits. Laboratory studies show that when individuals are subjected to stress, emotional support reduces the usual sharp rise in blood pressure and increased secretion of damaging stress-related hormones. One report demonstrated that middle-aged men who had recently endured high levels of emotional stress but had little social support were three times more likely to die over the next seven years. Lack of social support has been found to increase death rates following a heart attack and to delay recovery following cardiac surgery. Conversely, a happy marriage or good long-term relationship at age fifty was a leading indicator of being healthy at age eighty, whereas having a low cholesterol level had very little significance. Emotional support also reduces the risk of coronary events in individuals with Type A behavior.

Caregiver Stress

Sheila and I met when she attended a community presentation I was invited to deliver regarding Alzheimer's disease. She attended with her husband, who is in the early stages of Alzheimer's disease and also in a state of denial. The patient reluctantly agreed to have me provide care to him. I did find him in a complete state of denial regarding his memory impairment. It was difficult for me to get him to make return visits. Sheila appeared quite frustrated with his behavior, especially his belligerence toward me. She did convince him to continue to keep appointments with me, and I placed him on various medications in an attempt to improve his deteriorating cognitive state and his behavior. Unfortunately, none of this was particularly effective. There were side effects from these medications, so I withdrew them.

Significantly long gaps occurred between our visits. Sheila did her best to find support as a caregiver but this was limited. There was no family support at all. It was the second marriage for both, their children lived out of state, and they were resistant to becoming involved. The burden of providing care to her husband twenty-four hours a day seven days a week became excessive. As the pressure became unbearable, Sheila took an overdose of sleeping pills. A friend found her in the morning and got her to the hospital, thus saving her life.

With social service involvement, the situation improved for a while, but her husband's declining cognitive state continued to take a toll on her existence. Sheila would confide in me that she had a spineless existence. From the moment she got up in the morning and all day long, she provided care and supervision to her resistant husband. In the absence of a support system, she lived constantly on the edge of her breaking point.

An important sidebar topic to any discussion of stress and the aging is the impact it has on caregivers tasked with assisting or caring for someone who is ill or incapacitated.

Some studies suggest that caregivers—who often are on call for long hours or are required to support loved ones through painful crises—are also at risk of disruptions in their immune system function, as well as increased inflammation and frequent bouts of depression. Such individuals, regardless of their age, have weaker immune responses to vaccines, increased susceptibility to infection, and delayed wound healing. (103)

Inflammation is a normal response to injury and stress that is triggered by the production of chemicals such as interleukin-6. Too much inflammation has been implicated in several age-related diseases, including Alzheimer's and Parkinson's disease, arthritis, Type-2 diabetes and coronary heart disease. One study of men and women serving as caregivers to spouses with Alzheimer's disease found that they had a fourfold annual increase in interleukin-6 levels compared with age-matched controls without such responsibilities. What is particularly disturbing is that even when caregiving ceased due to the death of a spouse, increased interleukin-6 levels persisted for years. (104)

In another study, senior citizens who felt stressed out from taking care of their disabled spouses were sixty-three percent more likely to die within four years than caregivers without this complaint. And in a study that focused on telomere research, spouses and children who provided such constant care shortened their lives by as much as four to eight years. Caregivers also had double the rate of severe depression. (105)

Some of the early warning signs of caregiver stress are:

- Feeling overwhelmed, lonely, guilty, sad, or constantly worried
- Feeling fatigued most of the time
- Becoming easily irritated or angered
- Lack of interest in activities previously enjoyed
- Significant change in weight or sleep habits
- Frequent headaches, neck or low back pain
- Abuse of alcohol or drugs

In addition to the biological stress of just being alive, it is clear that we live in an age of additional stresses. We are living longer, but in a degraded and often unpeaceful environment, experiencing faster information loops and longer working hours. Research into the impact of stress on human physiology is growing by leaps and bounds, introducing much new knowledge about what can be done to mitigate the stress-related damage of growing older. In the section that follows, I'll share some tips and observations about dealing with stress GRACEfully.

S is for Stress—Formula
How to Achieve Balance and Peace

Raj was a very successful IT entrepreneur when he began seeing me as his Florida physician while spending half the year in this area. His parents were both of Indian descent and there was a family history of high blood pressure, diabetes, and high cholesterol. Since Raj was slender and he ate what he considered a healthy diet, he found it difficult to imagine that he could have high cholesterol and elevated blood pressure. Nonetheless, I tested him several times and found that, based on the guidelines we use to treat high blood pressure and high cholesterol, his diet and exercise program failed to get him to goal. Therefore, medication would be appropriate.

He has been a difficult patient who made it his business to tell me how to do my job and what to treat and what to ignore. He believed that he could just wish away his high BP and elevated cholesterol. Some of the problems he had were due to work and stress he had at home raising two active children and spending satisfactory time with his wife. He is certainly aware of the huge pressures he put upon himself to be successful at work. He intended to sell his business, and a great amount of money remained at stake. At the urging of his wife, he attended a week-long retreat to learn meditation techniques.

When he returned from the retreat he scheduled an immediate visit to my office. He had taken himself off all of his medication. Much to my amazement, his blood pressure was better. He told me about the type of retreat he went to. During that entire week, he learned in detail how to practice this form of meditation. He told me that the meditation would take two to three hours to do; at the end he was saturated with perspiration. He told me he felt wonderful and that he, his wife, and their children noticed substantial differences in his level of patience. Though he never told me of sleep issues beforehand, he was now sleeping better, waking up much more relaxed and refreshed. The meditation enabled him to think more clearly and make better business decisions.

In his words, he became "a new man."

Many years ago I became interested in understanding the scientific basis for meditation and relaxing, even though, at the time, I was skeptical about these "foreign" techniques. This was largely because I had discovered the book *Relaxation Response* by Herbert Benson, MD. I have referred to it often in the ensuing thirty years and have used to this day the techniques he describes in his book as my method of meditating. (106)

What I find fascinating about these exercises has to do with survival instincts. Animals, including humans, are hard-wired to defend themselves with a "fight or flight" reflex. When challenged, animals either fight their adversary or flee—an instantaneous survival mechanism. Similarly, animals, including humans, have to rest or recharge and change their brain waves, which is what happens during meditation. Benson has made a career of studying the techniques used by communities all over the world in the universal search for the health benefits of relaxation/meditation/mindfulness.

Meditation

Meditation is a mind-body practice with origins in ancient religious and spiritual traditions. The practice started thousands of years ago and first became popular in Asia with the teachings of Buddha, who practiced meditation himself. Eventually, the Buddhist form of meditation spread to the Western world, where it remains popular today. In meditation, one learns to focus attention while trying to eliminate or diffuse normal streams of thought. The practice is believed to result in a state of greater relaxation and mental calmness.

Meditation can be used as a mind-body medicine that generally focuses on two things: interactions between the brain, body, and behavior of an individual, and the ways in which emotional, mental, social, spiritual, and behavioral factors affect health. Meditation can be used to help reduce anxiety, pain, depression, stress, and insomnia. It can alleviate physical and emotional symptoms associated with chronic illnesses and their respective treatments. Meditation can also be used for overall wellness.

Here is more information about some of the popular techniques to use.

How Meditation Works

When our bodies are exposed to a sudden stress or threat, we respond with a characteristic "fight or flight" response. This is when epinephrine (adrenaline) and norepinephrine are released from the adrenal glands, resulting in an increase in blood pressure and pulse rate, faster breathing and increased blood flow to the muscles. Every time your body triggers the "fight or flight" response to a situation that is not life threatening, you are experiencing what is essentially a false alarm. Too many false alarms experienced by the body can lead to stress-related disorders such as heart disease, high blood pressure, migraine headaches, insomnia, sexual dysfunction and immune system disorders.

A simple meditation technique practiced for as few as ten minutes per day can help you control stress, decrease anxiety, improve cardiovascular health, and achieve greater capacity for relaxation.

The Relaxation Response

The technique referred to as The Relaxation Response has gained acceptance by physicians and therapists worldwide as a valuable adjunct to therapies for symptom relief in conditions ranging from cancer to AIDS. It was developed by Harvard Medical School physician Herbert Benson in the 1970s and is designed to elicit a state of deep relaxation in which breathing, pulse rate, blood pressure and metabolism are decreased. Training on a daily basis to achieve this state of relaxation can lead to enhanced mood, lowered blood pressure and a reduction of lifestyle stress.

The two essential steps to the relaxation response are:

- The repetition of a word, sound, phrase, prayer, or muscular activity.
- Passive disregard of everyday thoughts that inevitably come to mind during the process, followed by a return to the repetition.

To elicit the relaxation response:

- Choose a focus word or phrase for repetition. You can use a sound such as "ohm," a word such as "one" or "peace," or a word with special meaning to you.
- Sit in a comfortable position in a quiet place free of distractions. Close your eyes and relax your muscles progressing from your feet to your calves, thighs, abdomen, shoulders, head and neck.
- Breathe slowly and naturally and, as you do, say your focus word, sound, phrase or prayer silently to yourself while you exhale.
- To the best of your ability, dismiss intruding worries or thoughts by focusing on the repetition.

- Continue for ten to twenty minutes. It's okay to open your eyes to look at a clock while you are practicing, but do not set an alarm.
- When you have finished, remain seated, first with your eyes closed and then with your eyes open, and gradually allow your thoughts to return to everyday reality.

The Relaxation Response can also be elicited through other meditative and relaxation techniques. No matter how you achieve the relaxation state, regular practice can reduce the physical and emotional consequences of stress. (107)

Deep Breathing

This is one of the easiest stress management techniques to learn, and it can be done anywhere! When we become stressed, one of our body's automatic reactions is shallow, rapid breathing, which can increase our stress response. Taking deep, slow breaths is an antidote to stress and is one way we can "turn off" our stress reaction and "turn on" the relaxation response. Deep breathing is the foundation of many other relaxation exercises. Try this technique:

- Get into a comfortable position, either sitting or lying down.
- Put one hand on your stomach, just below your rib cage.
- Slowly breathe in through your nose. Your stomach should feel like it is rising and expanding outwards.
- Exhale slowly through your mouth, emptying your lungs completely and letting your stomach deflate.
- Repeat several times until you feel relaxed.
- Practice several times a day.

Information about The Relaxation Response is adapted from research by the Benson-Henry Institute for Mind Body Medicine.

Progressive Muscle Relaxation (PMR)

PMR is a technique for stress management developed by American physician Edmund Jacobson in the early 1920s. Jacobson argued that since muscular tension accompanies anxiety, an individual may reduce negative feelings by learning how to relax and relieve the muscular tension. (108)

PMR is based on alternately tensing and then relaxing the muscles. A person can practice this technique sitting or lying down in a comfortable spot. The key to the relaxation process is taking a few deep breaths and alternately tensing, then relaxing a group of muscles in systematic order. Focus on the head and scalp, move down to the neck, shoulders, etc., or start with the feet and legs and work up. The goal of the process is to promote deeper relaxation in the body than by simply attempting to relax.

A Simple Exercise to Help You Relax in Ten Steps

1. Sit in a comfortable position, with eyes closed. Take a few deep breaths, expanding your belly as you breathe air in, and contracting it as you exhale.
2. Begin at the top of your body and go down. Start with your head, tensing your facial muscles, squeezing your eyes shut, puckering your mouth and clenching your jaw. Hold, then release and breathe.
3. Tense as you lift your shoulders to your ears, hold, then release and breathe.
4. Make a fist with your right hand, then tighten the muscles in your lower and upper arm. Hold, then release. Breathe in and out. Repeat with left hand.
5. Concentrate on your back, squeezing shoulder blades together. Hold, then release. Breathe in and out.
6. Suck in your stomach, hold, then release. Breathe in and out.
7. Clench your buttocks. Hold, then release. Breathe in and out.
8. Tighten your right hamstring. Hold, then release. Breathe in and out. Repeat with left hamstring.
9. Flex your right calf muscle. Hold, then release. Breathe in and out. Repeat with left calf.
10. Tighten the toes on your right foot. Hold, then release. Breathe in and out. Repeat with the left foot.

This exercise is adapted from www.arthritistoday.org (109)

Caregiver Stress

Personal, employment and financial concerns are well established sources of stress in our society. There are countless resources for readers to address them, and it is beyond the scope of this book to try to do so. Caregiver stress is insidious in its onset, painful and not as popular as a subject of discussion. As a primary care physician and geriatrician who treats older adults and their baby boomer children, I see firsthand the ravages of this burden and therefore have chosen to include it in this book. Certainly the other sources of stress need attention and will benefit from taking action to alleviate them.

Caring for a loved one through an illness or decline can cause a special kind of stress. Nursing is hard enough (long hours, vigilance, lifting, and cleaning), but being emotionally involved with a patient can make it especially challenging. Full-time in-home care can relieve some of the stress of dealing with illness or infirmity within a couple or family, but that may not be part of everyone's financial reality.

Here are a few tips that may help you (or your caregiver!) cope with the particular stresses of the job:

- Try to lighten your load by learning about local caregiving resources such as meal delivery, home healthcare services (nursing, physical therapy), non-medical assistance (housekeeping, cooking, companionship) or home modification changes that make it easier for patients to bathe, use the toilet or move around.
- If your loved one is not bedridden and does not have dementia, emergency response systems (such as a call button on a necklace, bracelet, or belt they can wear) can alert medical personnel and you. You can use an intercom system to hear someone in another room, or a Webcam video camera to see him or her. Mobility monitors can keep track of dementia patients who wear a transmitter strapped to an ankle or wrist that will alert you when they move out of range.
- Make a list of your priorities (including those that pertain to your own wellbeing) and establish a daily routine.
- Try to find time to be physically active as much as possible, get enough sleep and eat properly.

- Make time each week to do something you enjoy and can look forward to, such as shopping or seeing a movie.
- Set realistic goals around household chores and administration by breaking large tasks into smaller ones you can do individually, as you have time.
- Stay in touch with family and friends but say "no" to requests that you no longer can easily handle, such as hosting holiday meals.
- If you need financial help taking care of a relative, don't be afraid to ask family members to contribute their fair share.
- Similarly, don't hesitate to ask for and accept assistance from others. Make a list of things that friends or family could help with. Let them choose what is best for them, such as assisting with meals, shopping for groceries, relieving you for a few hours, or taking the patient for a walk once or twice a week.
- Social support is a powerful stress buster, and in addition to family and friends, there may be a support group for caregivers in your situation. Joining one may allow you to make new friends and pick up useful tips from others who have had similar problems. Check with your local Area Agency on Aging (AAA) for information.

Stress is insidious. We all know about the emotional toll it takes on us psychologically but as I have detailed in this chapter it takes a tremendous toll on our bodies, contributing to disease and affecting the quality and duration of our lives.

Power of 5 Pointers
Chapter 4-Stress

1. Stress affects chemical processes in the human body leading to inflammation and premature aging.
2. Stress has the same negative effect on your body as does smoking and obesity.
3. Stress and the chemical changes and inflammation that result have been considered as possible contributors to neurodegenerative diseases such as Alzheimer's disease, Parkinson's disease, arthritis, diabetes, and coronary artery disease.
4. Addressing lifestyle concerns will reduce stress and the negative impact on one's health.
5. Techniques such as meditation, relaxation response and exercise offset the negative effects of stress.

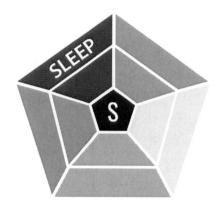

CHAPTER 5

SLEEP... "Good Night, Sleep Tight"; It will Save your Life

Sleep and sleep disorders were but a footnote in the medical education of the 1980s when I was training to be a geriatric physician. But I recall two experiences during my internship that I filed away for reference until I needed them thirty years later. Some details are fuzzy—for all I know the following experiences might have occurred within the same twenty-four-hour period of time.

I had been covering for another intern named David, who told me about a large African-American man in the intensive care unit. During the exchange of information session that happens every time one doctor takes over for another, David informed me that this man had been admitted to emergency with a hypertensive recording of blood pressure of 230/120. This is very bad, but he had been improving in the "unit." David added that the previous night the patient's blood pressure had abruptly gone up and he was given the medication Clonidine, which is known to be sedating. Shortly thereafter the patient stopped breathing and had to have an endotracheal tube threaded through his mouth into his lung in order to support his respirations. I was informed that this medicine would be used again if the patient's systolic blood pressure became elevated above 180. David advised me that I should be alert to the possibility of a repeat performance.

This might have been my first experience as a medical professional of the "you had it before and you got it again" phenomenon. Like clockwork, when the big, fat man fell asleep, his blood pressure went up and the nurse gave him the same sedating medication. I was paged to the intensive care unit where an endotracheal tube was again placed in the man's lungs to support his breathing. This was my first experience of sleep apnea, or what was then called "Pickwickian syndrome" and was probably the most extreme I would see for years. The entire experience left an indelible image in my brain.

My second experience may have occurred the next day. As a result of caring for the man with sleep apnea, I had had no more than two hours of sleep the prior night. I felt the same way I did the only time in my life I had too much to drink and experienced a hangover. I just couldn't get my brain to engage properly. At the end of that workday I made it home somehow, ate dinner, got into bed, and went off to sleep after experiencing my first case of sleep deprivation. It would not be my last.

I have never felt that I was putting a patient in jeopardy, but I have to admit that I had allowed myself to become deprived of sleep during that one period of my internship and residency. Ever since, I have taken strides to avoid it.

I worry about the extent of the sleep deprivation problem in our fast-paced, overworked and stressed society. Patients often come to their medical provider looking for the quick fix of sleeping pills to overcome what I now view as a medical condition. Here is a story about another one of my patients as an illustration.

I have known Alex for many years, but he became a patient only recently. Alex had always felt he was very healthy and avoided seeing a physician. Only at his wife's insistence did he become a patient of mine. He was thirty-five pounds over his ideal body weight and was no longer able to exercise much due to his work schedule, his finances and his arthritic knees. After his most recent exam, I became suspicious that he might have a sleep disorder such as sleep apnea. His waistline was forty-one-and-a-half inches indicative of his obesity and one of many risk factors for sleep apnea. When I looked at his throat, his uvula (the fleshy extension at the back of the soft palate) folded back onto his tongue, so I could not see the usual opening at the back of his throat that would allow air to flow easily into his lungs. He denied snoring, but his wife quickly corrected him.

When I suggested that Alex could have sleep apnea, he glared at me. When I offered to test him, he declined. An unwilling patient who finds he or she has sleep apnea and is quick to decline intervention presents a difficult situation for any primary care physician.

Six months later, after his wife brought him to the ER, I admitted Alex to the hospital for an overnight observation. In the week leading up to this event, Alex had been working late at night and getting up early to complete a project. The day before his ER visit, Alex drank two beers at lunch (an uncommon event for him) and when he awoke the day of his admission, he was unsteady on his feet. His wife noticed and was concerned. After numerous scans and blood tests, no abnormalities were detected and Alex was sent home.

During his follow-up visit I quizzed Alex about his sleeping habits over the previous few months. While he denied any change, his wife was very vocal in her concerns that Alex had not been himself. She had found him always very tired and even moody. When sleep testing was performed my suspicions were confirmed—Alex had moderate sleep apnea. The subsequent treatment resulted in a dramatic change that even Alex was forced to admit.

The National Institute of Neurological Disorders and Stroke reported the following on its website. (110) Nerve-signaling chemicals called neurotransmitters control whether we are asleep or awake by acting on different groups of nerve cells, or neurons, in the brain. Neurons in the brainstem, which connects the brain with the spinal cord, produce neurotransmitters such as serotonin and norepinephrine that keep some parts of the brain active while we are awake.

During sleep, we usually pass through five phases of sleep: stages one, two, three, four, and REM (rapid eye movement) sleep. These stages progress in a cycle from stage one to REM sleep, then the cycle starts over again with stage one.

We spend almost fifty percent of our total sleep time in stage two sleep, about twenty percent in REM sleep, and the remaining thirty percent in the other stages. Infants, by contrast, spend about half of their sleep time in REM sleep.

When we switch into REM sleep, our breathing becomes more rapid, irregular, and shallow, our eyes jerk rapidly in various directions, and our limb muscles become temporarily paralyzed. Our heart rate increases, our blood pressure rises, and males develop penile erections. When people awaken during REM sleep, they often describe bizarre and illogical tales—dreams. By morning, people spend nearly all their sleep time in stages one, two, and REM.

Since sleep and wakefulness are influenced by different neurotransmitter signals in the brain, foods and medicines that change the balance of these signals affect whether we feel alert or drowsy and how well we sleep. Caffeinated drinks such as coffee and drugs such as diet pills and decongestants stimulate some parts of the brain and can cause insomnia, or an inability to sleep. Many antidepressants suppress REM sleep. Heavy smokers often sleep very lightly and have reduced amounts of REM sleep. They also tend to wake up after three or four hours of sleep due to nicotine withdrawal. Many people who suffer from insomnia try to solve the problem with alcohol—the so-called nightcap. While alcohol does help people fall into light sleep, it also robs them of REM and the deeper, more restorative stages of sleep. Instead, it keeps them in the lighter stages of sleep, from which they can be awakened easily.

The amount of sleep each person needs depends on many factors, including age. For most adults, seven to eight hours a night appears to be the best amount. Getting too little sleep creates a "sleep debt," which is much like being overdrawn at a bank. Eventually, your body will demand that the debt be repaid. We don't seem to adapt to getting less sleep than we need; while we may get used to a sleep-depriving schedule, our judgment, reaction time, and other functions are still impaired. (111)

Researching the Link between Sleep Duration and Chronic Disease
Three main types of studies help us understand the links between sleep habits and the risk of developing certain diseases. The first type, called sleep deprivation studies, involves depriving healthy research volunteers of sleep and

examining any short-term physiological changes that could trigger disease. Such studies have revealed a variety of potentially harmful effects of sleep deprivation usually associated with increased stress, such as increased blood pressure, impaired control of blood glucose, and increased inflammation.

The second type of research, called cross-sectional epidemiological studies, involves interviewing subjects about their habitual sleep duration and the existence of a particular disease or group of diseases. For example, both reduced duration and increased sleep duration, as reported on questionnaires, are linked with hypertension, diabetes, and obesity. However, cross-sectional studies cannot explain how too little or too much sleep leads to disease. People may have a disease that affects sleep, rather than a sleep habit that causes a disease to occur or worsen.

The third and most convincing type of evidence that long-term sleep habits are associated with the development of numerous diseases comes from tracking sleep habits and disease patterns over long periods of time in individuals who are initially healthy. This tracking is called longitudinal epidemiological studies. We do not yet know whether adjusting one's sleep can reduce the risk of eventually developing a disease or lessen the severity of an ongoing disease. However, the results from longitudinal epidemiological studies are now beginning to suggest that this is likely.

Both animal and human research studies suggest that adequate sleep is crucial for a long and healthy life. Below are descriptions of some of the studies that look at the relationship between sleep habits and risk for developing certain medical conditions.

Obesity

Several studies have linked insufficient sleep and weight gain. For example, studies have shown that people who habitually sleep less than six hours per night are much more likely to have a higher than average body mass index (BMI) and that people who sleep eight hours have the lowest BMI. Lack of sleep is now being seen as a potential risk factor for obesity along with the two other most commonly identified risk factors: lack of exercise and overeating. Research into the mechanisms involved in regulating metabolism and appetite begins to explain what might be the connection between sleep and obesity.

During sleep, our bodies secrete hormones that help to control appetite, energy metabolism, and glucose processing. Glucose, you may recall, is the high-energy carbohydrate that cells use for fuel. Obtaining too little sleep upsets the balance of these and other hormones. For example, poor sleep leads to an increase in the production of cortisol, as you have learned, often referred to as the "stress hormone." Poor sleep is also associated with increases in the secretion of insulin following a meal. As you learned earlier in this book, insulin is a hormone that regulates glucose processing and promotes fat storage; higher levels of insulin are associated with weight gain, a risk factor for diabetes.

Insufficient sleep is also associated with lower levels of leptin, the hormone that alerts the brain that it has enough food, as well as higher levels of ghrelin, a biochemical that stimulates appetite. As a result, poor sleep may result in food cravings, even after we have eaten an adequate number of calories. We may also be more likely to eat foods such as sweets that satisfy the craving for a quick energy boost. In addition, insufficient sleep may leave us too tired to burn off these extra calories with exercise.

Diabetes

Researchers have found that insufficient sleep may lead to Type-2 diabetes by influencing the way the body processes glucose. One short-term sleep restriction study found that a group of healthy subjects who had their sleep cut back from eight to four hours per night processed glucose more slowly than they did when they were permitted to sleep for twelve hours. Numerous epidemiological studies also have revealed that adults who usually slept less than five hours per night have a greatly increased risk of having or developing diabetes.

I'll discuss this very serious medical condition and its intersection with sleep hygiene further in the chapter.

Heart Disease and Hypertension

Studies have found that a single night of inadequate sleep in people who have existing hypertension can cause elevated blood pressure throughout the following day. This effect may begin to explain the correlation between poor sleep and cardiovascular disease and stroke. For example, one study found that sleeping too little—less than six hours—or too much—more than nine hours—increased the risk of coronary heart disease in women.

There is also growing evidence of a connection between obstructive sleep apnea and heart disease. Over time, this condition can lead to chronic hypertension, which is a major risk factor for cardiovascular disease. Fortunately, when sleep apnea is treated, blood pressure often goes down.

I'll take a closer look at the connection between disrupted sleep and heart disease later in the chapter.

Mood Disorders

Given that a single sleepless night can cause people to be irritable and moody the following day, it is conceivable that chronic insufficient sleep may lead to long-term mood disorders. Chronic sleep issues have been correlated with depression, anxiety, and mental distress. In one study, subjects who slept four and a half hours per night reported feeling more stressed, sad, angry, and mentally exhausted. In another study, subjects who slept four hours per night showed declining levels of optimism and sociability as one result of days of inadequate sleep. All of these self-reported symptoms improved dramatically when subjects returned to a normal eight-hour sleep schedule.

More on this later in the chapter.

Immune Function

It is natural for people to go to bed when they are sick. Substances produced by the immune system to help fight infection also cause fatigue. One theory proposes that the immune system evolved "sleepiness-inducing factors" because inactivity and sleep provided an advantage: those who slept more when faced with an infection were better able to fight that infection than those who slept less. Research in animals suggests that animals that obtain more deep sleep following experimental challenge by microbial infection have a better chance of survival.

Alcohol

As mentioned previously, despite its mild sedative qualities, alcohol often contributes to poor sleep. Studies have shown that alcohol use is more prevalent among people who sleep poorly. It is best to avoid or eliminate alcohol consumption if sleeping is disrupted or inadequate.

Sleep and Life Expectancy

Considering the many potential adverse health effects of insufficient sleep, it is not surprising that poor sleep is associated with lower life expectancy. Data from three large cross-sectional epidemiological studies reveal that sleeping five hours or less per night increased mortality risk from all causes by roughly fifteen percent. (112)

Of course, just as sleep problems can affect disease risk, several diseases and disorders can also affect the amount of sleep we get. While an estimated fifty to seventy million Americans suffer from some type of sleep disorder, most people do not mention sleeping problems to their doctors, and most doctors do not routinely ask about them. This widespread lack of awareness of the impact of sleep problems can have serious and costly public health consequences. Those individuals who experience disturbed sleep for any reason should seek help from a medical provider. Your overall health and wellbeing are at stake.

Living GRACEFULLY includes attention paid to sleep hygiene, as well as all other aspects of your life.

Sleep Disorders

At least forty million Americans suffer from chronic long-term sleep disorders each year, and an additional twenty million experience occasional sleeping problems. These disorders and the resulting sleep deprivation interfere with work, driving, and social activities. They also account for an estimated $16 billion in medical costs each year, while the indirect costs due to lost productivity and other factors are probably much greater. Doctors have described more than seventy sleep disorders, most of which can be managed effectively once they are correctly diagnosed. The most common sleep disorders include insomnia, sleep apnea, restless legs syndrome, and narcolepsy. In many of the sleep disorders mentioned, there is a disruption in sleep cycles. As previously noted, the rapid eye movement (REM or dream) portion of sleep is particularly important. When it is disrupted, there are major consequences in brain function and activity. Loss of this component leads to loss of concentration and can have negative implications on our metabolism and hormonal mechanisms. (113)

Insomnia

Almost everyone occasionally suffers from short-term insomnia. Problems can result from stress, jet lag, diet, and many other factors. Insomnia almost always affects job performance and well-being, especially the day after a restless night.

About sixty million Americans per year have insomnia frequently or for extended periods of time. Simple insomnia can lead to even more serious sleep deficits. Insomnia tends to increase with age, starting in our late teenage years, and worsens over time. Insomnia affects about forty percent of women and thirty percent of men. It is often the major disabling symptom of an underlying medical disorder. (114)

For short-term insomnia, doctors may prescribe sleeping pills. Most sleeping pills stop working after several weeks of nightly use, however, and long-term use can create dependency, and can actually interfere with good sleep. Mild insomnia often can be prevented or cured by practicing good sleep habits. See *Basic* **Tips for a Good Night's Sleep** at the end of this chapter. For more serious cases of insomnia, researchers are experimenting with light therapy and other ways to alter circadian cycles—the twenty-four-hour physiological cycle of most living beings. It can be modulated by things like light and temperature.

Sleep Apnea

Sleep apnea is a disorder that results in interrupted breathing during sleep. (Remember my intern experiences described earlier in the chapter?) It usually occurs in conjunction with the fat buildup or loss of muscle tone that comes with aging. These changes allow the windpipe to collapse during breathing when muscles relax during sleep. *Obstructive sleep apnea* is usually associated with loud snoring, although not everyone who snores has the disorder. Sleep apnea can also occur if the neurons that control breathing malfunction during sleep.

During an episode of obstructive apnea, the person's effort to inhale air creates suction that collapses the windpipe. This can block airflow for ten seconds up to a minute while the sleeping person struggles to breathe. When the person's blood oxygen level falls, the brain responds by waking the person just enough to tighten the upper airway muscles and open the windpipe. The person may snort or gasp, then resume snoring. This cycle may be repeated hundreds of times a night.

The frequent awakenings that sleep apnea patients experience can leave them continually sleepy and may lead to personality changes such as irritability or depression. Sleep apnea also deprives the person of oxygen. Such deprivation can lead to morning headaches, a loss of interest in sex, or a decline in mental functioning. It is linked to high blood pressure, irregular heartbeats, and an increased risk of heart attacks and stroke. Patients with severe, untreated sleep apnea are two to three times more likely to have automobile accidents than the general population. In some high-risk individuals, sleep apnea may even lead to sudden death from respiratory arrest during sleep.

An estimated eighteen million Americans have sleep apnea. However, few of them have had the problem diagnosed. Patients who exhibit the typical features of sleep apnea, such as loud snoring, obesity and excessive daytime sleepiness, should be referred to a specialized sleep center that can perform a test called *polysomnography* ; also known as a sleep study. This test records the patient's brain waves, heartbeat and breathing during an entire night. If sleep apnea is diagnosed, several treatments are available. Mild sleep apnea can often be overcome through weight loss, or by preventing the person from sleeping on his or her back. Other sufferers may need special devices or surgery to correct the obstruction. People with sleep apnea should never take sedatives or sleeping pills, which can prevent them from awakening enough to breathe. In other words, they could suffer severe injury to their nervous system. They could even die.

Restless Legs Syndrome

Restless legs syndrome (RLS) is a familial disorder causing unpleasant crawling, prickling or tingling sensations in the legs and feet and an urge to move them for relief. It is emerging as one of the most common sleep disorders, especially among older people, often starting after age fifty. The disorder, which affects as many as twelve million Americans, leads to constant leg movement during the day and insomnia at night. Severe RLS is most common in elderly people, though symptoms may develop at any age. In some cases, it may be linked to other conditions such as anemia, pregnancy, or diabetes.

Many RLS patients also have a disorder known as *periodic limb movement disorder* or PLMD, which causes repetitive jerking movements of the limbs, especially the legs. These movements occur every twenty to forty seconds and can cause repeated awakening and severely fragmented sleep. In one study, RLS and PLMD accounted for a third of the insomnia seen in patients older than age sixty.

Drugs that affect the neurotransmitter dopamine can relieve both RLS and PLMD, suggesting that dopamine abnormalities may underlie the symptoms exhibited by sufferers of these conditions. Learning how these disorders occur may lead to better therapies in the future.

Narcolepsy

Narcolepsy affects an estimated 250,000 Americans. People with narcolepsy have frequent "sleep attacks," suddenly falling fast asleep at various times of the day, even if they have had a normal amount of sleep during the night. These attacks can last from several seconds to more than thirty minutes. People with narcolepsy also may experience cataplexy (loss of muscle control during emotional situations), hallucinations and temporary paralysis when they awaken, in addition to disrupted nighttime sleep. These symptoms seem to resemble common features of REM sleep that can appear when a person wakes suddenly. Their appearance suggests that narcolepsy is a disorder of sleep regulation.

Symptoms of narcolepsy typically appear during adolescence, though it often takes years to obtain a correct diagnosis. The disorder, or at least a predisposition to it, is usually hereditary, but occasionally it is linked to brain damage from a head injury or neurological disease.

Once narcolepsy is diagnosed, stimulants, antidepressants, or other drugs can help control the symptoms and prevent the embarrassing and dangerous effects of falling asleep at improper times. Naps at certain times of the day may also reduce excessive daytime sleepiness.

Sleep research is expanding, currently attracting more and more attention from scientists. Researchers now know that sleep is an active and dynamic state that greatly influences our waking hours, and they realize that we must understand sleep to fully understand the brain. Innovative techniques, such as brain imaging, can now help researchers understand how different brain regions function during sleep and how different activities and disorders affect sleep. Understanding the factors that affect sleep in health and disease also may lead to revolutionary new therapies for sleep disorders and to ways of overcoming jet lag and the problems associated with shift work. We can expect these and many other benefits from research that will allow us to truly understand sleep's impact on our lives.

Existing Medical Conditions That May Lead to Disturbed Sleep

In addition to the conditions described above, there are a great many additional causes for disturbed sleep and/or poor sleep quality. Some are related to existing or undiagnosed medical and mental health conditions, and some have even been linked to the use of prescription and over-the-counter medication. (See my medication table later in the chapter.)

Conditions commonly associated with sleep problems include heartburn, diabetes, cardiovascular disease, musculoskeletal disorders, kidney disease, mental health problems, neurological disorders, respiratory problems, and thyroid disease. Let's look a bit closer at each of these often chronic conditions.

Lying down in bed often worsens **heartburn**, a form of indigestion that is caused by the backup of stomach acid into the esophagus. One can avoid this problem by abstaining from heavy or fatty foods—as well as coffee and alcohol—during the evening. People suffering with this condition can also use gravity to their advantage by elevating the upper body with an under-mattress wedge or blocks placed under the bedposts. Over-the-counter and prescription drugs that suppress stomach acid secretion may also help.

Diabetes is a common and chronic disorder marked by elevated levels of blood glucose or sugar. People with diabetes whose blood sugar levels are not well controlled may experience sleep problems due to:

- night sweats
- a frequent need to urinate
- symptoms of hypoglycemia (low blood sugar)

If diabetes has damaged nerves in the legs, nighttime movements or pain may also disturb sleep.

Heart failure is a condition characterized by a gradual decline in the heart's ability to circulate blood adequately. Heart failure can cause fluid to build up in the lungs and tissues. Patients with heart failure may awaken during the night feeling short of breath because extra body fluid accumulates around their lungs when they're lying down. Using pillows to elevate the upper body may help. These people can also be awakened just as they are falling asleep by a characteristic breathing pattern called Cheyne-Stokes respiration, a series of increasingly deep breaths followed by a brief cessation of breathing.

Benzodiazepine sleep medications (the most commonly prescribed sleep medication in the U.S) help some people to stay asleep despite this kind of breathing disturbance, but others may need to use supplementary oxygen or a device that increases pressure in the upper airway and chest cavity to help them breathe and sleep more normally.

Men with heart failure frequently have obstructive sleep apnea (see above), which can disrupt sleep, cause daytime sleepiness and accelerate heart failure. For people with coronary artery disease, natural fluctuations in circadian rhythms may trigger angina (chest pain), arrhythmia (irregular heartbeat), or even heart attack while they are asleep.

Arthritis pain and other musculoskeletal disorders can make it hard for people to fall asleep and to resettle when they shift positions. In addition, pain relief treatment with steroids frequently causes insomnia. Taking aspirin or a non-steroidal anti-inflammatory drug (NSAID) just before bedtime is an effective alternative for relieving pain and swelling in the joints during the night.

People with **fibromyalgia,** a condition characterized by painful ligaments and tendons, are likely to wake in the morning still feeling fatigued and stiff. Researchers who analyzed the sleep of fibromyalgia sufferers have found that at least half have abnormal deep sleep. These patients exhibit slow brain waves that are mixed with waves usually associated with relaxed wakefulness – this abnormal pattern is called alpha-delta sleep. I have long believed that fibromyalgia is almost always linked to sleep disorders.

People with **kidney disease** have kidneys that are damaged to the extent that they can no longer filter fluids, remove wastes, and keep electrolytes in balance as efficiently as they did when healthy. Kidney disease can cause waste products to build up in the blood and can result in insomnia or symptoms of restless legs syndrome. Although researchers aren't sure why, kidney dialysis or transplant does not always return sleep to normal.

Nocturia is the need to get up frequently to urinate during the night. It is a common cause of sleep loss, especially among older adults. A mild case can cause a person to wake up at least twice during the night; in severe cases, a person may get up as many as five or six times. This condition may be a product of age, but other causes include medical conditions (heart failure, diabetes, urinary tract infection, an enlarged prostate, liver failure, multiple sclerosis, sleep apnea), medication (especially diuretics), and excessive fluid intake after dinner. Therapies for nocturia fall into three categories:

- treatments to correct medical causes
- behavioral interventions
- medication

The first step is to try to identify the cause and correct it. If this is unsuccessful, behavioral approaches such as cutting down on fluids in the two hours before bedtime (especially caffeine and alcohol) may be implemented. If the nocturia persists, doctors may prescribe one of a growing number of medications approved to treat an overactive bladder. Treatment of the sleep disorder is another important consideration which is often overlooked by physicians.

An **overactive thyroid gland** (hyperthyroidism) can also cause sleep problems. The disorder over-stimulates the nervous system, making it hard for the patient to fall asleep. It may cause night sweats, leading to nighttime arousals. Feeling cold and sleepy is a hallmark of an underactive thyroid (hypothyroidism). Because thyroid function affects every organ and system in the body, the symptoms can be wide-ranging and sometimes difficult to decipher. Checking thyroid function requires a simple blood test. Patients who notice a variety of unexplained symptoms can request a thyroid test from their physician.

The **breathing difficulties** that arise from several medical conditions can disturb sleep. Normal circadian-related changes in the tone of the muscles surrounding the airways can cause the airways to constrict during the night, raising the potential for nocturnal asthma attacks that rouse the sleeper abruptly. The fear of having an attack may make it more difficult to fall asleep, as can the use of steroids or other breathing medications that also have a stimulating effect similar to that of caffeine. People who have emphysema or bronchitis may also have difficulty falling and staying asleep because of excess sputum production, shortness of breath, and coughing.

Psychological Causes for Poor Sleep

Almost all people with anxiety or depression have trouble falling asleep and staying asleep. In turn, not being able to sleep may become a focus of some sufferers' ongoing fear and tension, causing further sleep loss.

Marie is one of my favorite patients. She is a feisty, slender Italian woman with light blond hair. (Only your hairdresser knows for sure). Although she has been generally healthy, over the years I have had to see her for many different medical problems. I have gotten to know what makes her tick and the emotional challenges she faces day in and day out. She has told me, "I care deeply about my children and grandchildren, but they live out of state and I am not able to visit them as often as I would like. My husband is a workaholic, so I don't get to spend as much time with him as I would like. I worry about everything and I have trouble sleeping at night. My blood pressure goes out of sight each time there is a crisis."

She has asked for my help on multiple occasions, but she never responded to my conservative suggestions of stress management or meditation. We have agreed to intermittent use of antianxiety medication that she can use during crisis situations and to help her sleep on her really bad nights.

Emotional stresses such as Marie has struggled with can be disruptive to normal sleep cycles. Grief is another good example of an emotional stress, as neurotransmitter balance is disrupted and the mind cannot turn itself off, with resulting disruption of our normal sleep cycles.

Here are descriptions of some of the most common and easy-to-treat sleep-disturbing psychological conditions. Consulting and partnering with a physician can result in phenomenal improvement in sleep and quality of life. Each of the examples that follows might be responsive to medication or another form of therapy that would be worth exploring.

General anxiety

Severe anxiety, also known as generalized anxiety disorder, is characterized by persistent, nagging feelings of worry, apprehension, or uneasiness. These feelings are either unusually intense or out of proportion to the real troubles and dangers of the person's everyday life. People with general anxiety typically experience excessive, persistent worry every day or almost every day for a period of six months or more. Common symptoms include trouble falling asleep, trouble staying asleep, and not feeling rested after sleep.

Depression

Because almost ninety percent of people with serious depression experience insomnia, a physician evaluating a person with insomnia will almost always consider depression as a possible cause. Waking up too early in the morning is a hallmark of depression, and some depressed people have difficulty falling asleep or they experience only fitful sleep throughout the whole night. In chronic, low-grade depression—also known as dysthymia—insomnia or sleepiness may be the most prominent symptom. Laboratory studies have shown that people who are depressed spend less time in slow-wave sleep and may enter REM sleep more quickly at the beginning of the night. The result is an inadequate amount of restorative sleep, which can result in imbalance in important neurotransmitters and persistent depression.

Bipolar disorder

Disturbed sleep is a prominent feature of bipolar disorder, also known as manic-depressive illness. Sleep loss may exacerbate or induce manic symptoms or it may temporarily alleviate depression. During a manic episode, a person may not sleep at all for several days. Such occurrences are often followed by a "crash" during which the person spends most of the next few days in bed.

Schizophrenia

Some people with schizophrenia sleep very little in the early, most severe stage of an episode. Between episodes, their sleep patterns are likely to improve, although many people with schizophrenia rarely obtain a normal amount of deep sleep.

Neurological Disorders and Disturbed Sleep

Certain brain and nerve disorders can contribute to sleeplessness.

Peter is a retired engineer of very high intellect. He has been suffering with a form of dementia called Lewy body dementia. His loss of intellectual capacity had been understandably very distressing to him. He tells me, "It is very depressing to suffer the loss of my capacity. I just cannot think of things the way I used to. I wake up at three a.m. and cannot turn my brain off and am frustrated that I cannot sleep. I get up and start bothering my wife, who needs her sleep. I just cannot help myself. I cannot cope when this happens in the middle of the night."

Peter's situation describes a fairly common phenomenon that individuals with dementia face.

Dementia

Alzheimer's disease and other forms of dementia may disrupt sleep regulation and other brain functions. Wandering, disorientation and agitation during the evening and night, a phenomenon known as "sundowning," can require constant supervision and place great stress on caregivers. In such cases, small doses of antipsychotic medications are more helpful than benzodiazepine drugs. It is important for this condition to be recognized and treated, as two or more people are affected. First is the individual who suffers from the condition and who is not getting restorative sleep and whose condition will worsen. In addition, the spouse or caregiver must be awake and alert enough to provide supervision and care. Without a well-rested caregiver there is a higher risk for adverse experiences for both the demented individual and the caregiver.

Epilepsy
People with epilepsy—a condition in which a person is prone to seizures—are twice as likely as others to suffer from insomnia. Brain wave disturbances that cause seizures can also cause deficits in slow-wave sleep or REM sleep. Anti-seizure drugs can cause similar changes at first, but tend to correct these sleep disturbances when used over time. About one in four people with epilepsy have seizures that occur at night, causing disturbed sleep and daytime sleepiness. Sleep deprivation can also trigger a seizure, a phenomenon noted in college infirmaries during exam periods, as some students suffer their first seizures after staying up late to study.

Headaches
People who are prone to headaches should try to practice good sleep hygiene, as lack of sleep can promote headaches. A tendency to both cluster headaches and migraines may be related to the increased susceptibility to changes in the size of the blood vessels leading to the cortex of the brain; pain occurs when the walls of the blood vessels dilate, caused by sleep deprivation. Another theory has to do with the release of certain proteins that cause pain that are prevalent in patients who experience sleep deprivation

Parkinson's disease
Almost all people with Parkinson's disease have insomnia. As the disease impacts motor function, just getting in and out of bed can be a struggle, and the disease often disrupts sleep. Some arousals are caused by the tremors and

movements caused by the disorder, and others seem to result from the disorder itself. As a result, daytime sleepiness is common.

Treatment with sleeping pills may be difficult because some drugs can worsen Parkinson's symptoms. Some patients who take drugs used to treat Parkinson's may develop severe nightmares; others experience disruption of REM sleep. However, the use of these medications at night is important to maintain the mobility needed to change positions in bed. A bed rail or an overhead bar—known as a trapeze—may make it easier for people with Parkinson's to move about and, therefore, lead to better sleep.

Consequences of Disrupted Sleep

The cost of poor sleep is much greater than many people think: it may have profound consequences for our long-term health. Research reveals that people who consistently fail to get enough sleep are at an increased risk of chronic medical conditions such as diabetes, high blood pressure, and heart disease. Additional research studies show that habitually sleeping more than nine hours is also associated with poor health. Treating sleep as a priority, rather than a luxury, may be as important a step as following a healthy diet in preventing a number of chronic medical conditions and preserving general mental and physical wellbeing.

S is for Sleep—Formula
The Essential Benefits of Rest and Repair

You've read my thoughts about clinical sleep disorders in the previous section. Many of us can periodically suffer from sleep disruptions that may easily be addressed through better habits related to sleeping routines. Though modern life makes it tempting to fill our most private rooms with gadgets and digital toys, the bedroom should be a calm place for relaxation, sleep, intimacy and nothing else. That includes television and computers.

Consider the following tips for achieving good sleep hygiene. Keep in mind that if you don't fall asleep within fifteen or twenty minutes, don't just stay in bed "trying harder" to drift off. You may need to further adjust some of your habits.

Create a haven for sleep

Your bedroom should be cool, dark, quiet and uncluttered. The recommended room temperature for sleeping is 61-65F. This is because a cooler body optimizes the release of the sleep hormone, melatonin. Blackout blinds are a sensible investment, as twenty percent of light can still reach the eyes through closed eyelids. If you are being awakened by noises, try earplugs. Keep your bedroom tidy and avoid working there. This room should be a calm place associated with, above all else, relaxation and sleep.

Banish blue light

Strategically located night-lights allow you to move around safely in the dark, but they have a drawback. They emit normal white light, which contains all the colors of the spectrum, including the energizing blue that makes it harder to get back to sleep. Invest in a specially designed night-light that cuts out the blue part of the spectrum, or use a low-blue bulb in an existing fitting.

Compensate for aging eyes

As we age, cataracts may begin to form and pupils may become smaller, reducing the amount of light reaching the retina and hampering the body's ability to recognize when we should be asleep or awake. Compensate for this by exposing yourself to more bright light during the day. Stop two or three hours before bedtime, to avoid interfering with the onset of nighttime melatonin production. Melatonin is a neurotransmitter released in the brain that promotes sleep. There are many other neurotransmitters in our brains that promote wakefulness. Under normal circumstances, they have a well-established balance that promotes sleep at night and wakefulness in the morning.

Work with your sleeping partner

Dealing with individual differences in sleep patterns requires compromise and consideration. If you prefer the cold, but your partner is a heat-seeker, he or she might have to consider wearing warmer nightwear in a cooler bedroom. If you are a night owl, but your partner is a morning lark, discuss ways of sharing the bedroom to prevent the disruption of each other's sleep patterns. Separate bedrooms can solve extreme differences, but talking constructively could lead to a solution that suits you both.

Check your sleeping posture

We spend a third of our lives in a sleeping posture and it should be our most restorative. You can't correct your posture while asleep, but you can buy the right mattress and pillow first, and then tackle any specific areas of discomfort. Replace your mattress after about eight years, and ignore the myth that hard mattresses are best; everything depends on your size and sleeping position. Take note of any beds in which you sleep well and consider buying the same type or brand.

Once you have the right mattress, fine-tune your sleeping position with extra pillows. If you sleep on your side, for example, putting a pillow between your knees will minimize any twisting strain on your lower back. If you have hip pain, a padded, sheepskin, or memory-foam mattress topper will help soften and contour things.

Find the perfect pillow

A woman with great posture who sleeps on her back may not need a pillow, while a large male side-sleeper may need two or three. Synthetic pillows should be replaced every six months to a year, down and feather pillows every two to five years. Sleeping on an old or inappropriately large or hard pillow can lead to discomfort and/or recurring neck and shoulder problems.

Three key questions to consider before buying a pillow:

- What is your favored sleeping position?
- How big are you?
- What is your personal preference?

Keep to a regular sleeping schedule

Go to bed and get up at roughly the same times each day to keep your body clock on track and promote your natural drive to sleep. Getting up at a similar time each morning is most important since lie-ins make it harder to get to sleep the next night.

Start noticing what times you feel and perform at your best, when you naturally wake without an alarm clock, and when you start to feel sleepy in the evenings. Once you know your "chronotype" (this terms refers to an individual's propensity for maximum wakefulness at a certain time of day), you can set healthy sleep goals that work with your natural circadian rhythms. A free online assessment at the Center for Environmental Therapeutics

(www.cet-surveys.com/index.php?sid=61524&newtest=Y) can help you find your type, and provide related advice.

Most people have inner clocks that run on a cycle of about twenty-four hours. But some people's rhythms may be an hour or more off the solar cycle—the cycle places the working day within daylight hours—making it harder for them to be alert when they need to be. Keep your circadian rhythms in sync with society by making sure you are exposed to light at the times of day most useful to your chronotype. Sunlight can be enough, but you may also like to consider bright-light therapy.

Healthy day, healthy night

Having a healthy lifestyle tends to lead to good-quality sleep, but there are two changes that could make a big difference. The first is limiting your caffeine intake to the morning and early afternoon. The stimulant stays in your system much longer than you might think and not only undermines sleep quality but can also exacerbate certain sleep disorders. Secondly, avoid excess alcohol, especially later in the evening. Although it can help you get to sleep, as the effects of alcohol wear off during the night, sleep becomes lighter or interrupted.

Similarly, timing your physical exercise can result in more effective release of chemicals and hormones that produce sleep of a better quality. One of the best times to exercise to improve sleep is in the late afternoon. However, vigorous exercise within three or four hours of bedtime can actually interfere with your sleep, since it raises the body's temperature, adrenalin levels, heart rate, and brain activity.

Wind down properly

If you can't sleep because your brain is whizzing, make an effort to disengage from the outside world an hour or two before bedtime. Stop working, come off social media, stop surfing the net, and try more relaxing activities such as chatting or having a bath. You could do a "mental download." To put your brain into neutral, write down everything that is whirring around in your head. But use a notebook and pen, NOT the computer. The screen of your computer is designed to be bright. That's fine during daylight hours, but it becomes unhealthy when bedtime is approaching because it fools your body into thinking you need to stay up. **F.lux**, a free app available at www.justgetflux.com, makes the color of your computer screen resemble the current time of day, helping your body recognize that bedtime is drawing near.

Snack on snooze foods

Turkey and warm milk contain tryptophan (the precursor to melatonin), while honey contains the neuropeptide orexin (also called hypocretin), which reduces alertness. Marmite, almonds, chamomile and oatcakes are also good, and bananas have high levels of serotonin and magnesium. Never go to bed hungry; try eating an early evening meal followed by a sleep-inducing bedtime snack several hours later.

Follow the twenty-minute rule

If you don't fall asleep within fifteen or twenty minutes, don't stay in bed "trying harder" to drift off. Instead, get out of bed; leave the bedroom and do something quiet and not stimulating, such as reading a book or knitting, until you feel sleepy again. The longer you toss and turn in bed, the more frustrated and anxious you will become and the longer it will take you to relax, unwind and, eventually, sleep.

Start a sleep diary

Sometimes we are unaware of bad habits until they are pointed out to us. A sleep diary, a smart phone app, or some other device such as a Fitbit can help us discover factors leading to poor sleep, as well as track treatments or behavior changes that are helping us sleep better. Complete your diary every morning, looking back over the past day and night. List each complete hour you were asleep in bed, and each partial hour (including naps). Then list events that may have influenced your sleep: drinking alcohol or caffeine, taking sleeping pills, exercising, eating, or using the washroom during the night, and when the event happened. Keep the diary for two weeks.

Be mindful of your thoughts and emotions

Many who struggle to sleep worry about the past—how little sleep they have had—and the future—how bad things will be if they don't sleep. Such worry only increases nighttime arousal and cultivates a "learned response," with the brain repeating the pattern of anxiety each night. Mindfulness—the practice of focusing on the present moment—has been shown to increase the speed at which people fall asleep and the quality of their sleep. Practice observing and letting go of your thoughts, and use your senses to notice the touch of the duvet on your toes, or the rise and fall of your breathing. Mindfulness allows you to observe fearful thoughts or strong sensations such as anxiety, but to become familiar with these thoughts and even welcome them. Try to achieve an objective view of thoughts by gently acknowledging them, rather than remaining trapped inside them.

The fear of not sleeping can drive some to place extreme controls on their lives: avoiding going out at night, being less ambitious at work, or sleeping in the spare room. This is not only dangerous but also futile, since extreme behavior only increases anxiety. Commit to making small actions every day that take you closer to what is important to you. A content brain is a sleepy brain. Don't battle with sleep; doing so will only wake you up further. Only by adopting an accepting attitude to wakefulness—letting go of the fight—can you bring the mental and physical peace that allows sleep to emerge naturally.

Consider alternative therapies

For sleep problems related to lifestyle, anecdotal evidence indicates that therapies such as acupuncture, homoeopathic remedies and massage may be useful.

As long as the treatment is not harmful, it may be worth trying. Of the many herbal preparations that claim to aid sleep, the flowering plant valerian has the most medical and scientific evidence supporting its effectiveness.

A final word on sleep disorders
It seems like once a week I have a patient in my office just like the following.

> Rachael is an eighty-one-year-old woman (but I have seen patients like this in their fifties) who during her initial visit described herself as "a retired know-it-all nurse." She came to see me when her former physician had retired. I am well acquainted with this physician and know he practices quality medicine. I have noticed sometimes when there is great familiarity between doctor and patient subtleties can be lost. At our initial visit she told me that she had been treated for high blood pressure. She added, "The medicine has worked very well and I am pleased that there are no side effects. I have concerns because lately I have been more tired than usual and find myself taking afternoon naps. In addition when I get up in the morning my bed is a mess, sheets everywhere and I never feel refreshed."
>
> "Do you snore?" I asked.
>
> She responded in a somewhat agitated fashion. "How should I know? My husband is nearly deaf, has dementia, and is asleep before me."
>
> At this point I scratched my head as if I had a lot to consider but I really didn't. I had a high suspicion that she had sleep apnea. I proceeded to ask a few more questions so she would not think my job was easy. I did a thorough exam; focusing on her neck size and her throat. When I had completed my work I said, "Rachael, I think you might have sleep apnea."
>
> She looked at me with horror and disbelief. "Doctor, are you out of your mind? I don't have sleep apnea, but I will do whatever tests you ask me to do as long as you can fix me."
>
> I'll cut to the chase. She was immensely cooperative with all the tests I put her through to get the proper diagnosis. She did, in fact, have sleep apnea. After I got her hooked up to a CPAP machine with the correct pressure, she came back for her scheduled office visit and with a great big hug and said, "Doctor, you were right, I do have sleep apnea

and now that I am using that stupid machine I have my life back. I am no longer snoring, I do not need to take an afternoon nap, and I wake up refreshed every day. In addition, I know this sounds stupid, but most importantly when I wake up in the morning my bed is neat and tidy and I barely have to fix the covers to get it made properly. Thank you. I should never have doubted you."

Sleep disorders have become very commonplace and well known in our society. Sleep disruption is a common subject of discussion amongst the baby boomer population, although no one wants to admit they suffer from it. Many patients who come to my office for a first visit have such obvious cases of sleeplessness that I jokingly say I can make the diagnosis of obstructive sleep apnea before I sit down in the room. Don't get me wrong. I do take a very thorough patient history and perform a complete exam. But really, the challenge comes in presenting my diagnosis and plan to the disbelieving patient. The implementation phase of a treatment plan is usually difficult as well.

Treatment of sleep apnea starts with recommendations for lifestyle modifications that include avoidance of alcohol and the taking of sedating medications. In addition, patients are advised to avoid esophageal reflux by not eating before bedtime. In some cases, patients are provided with a CPAP (continuous positive airway pressure) machine. This can provide a life altering modification, usually in a good way. I have seen firsthand the transformation that occurs when sleep apnea is correctly treated, and it is a gratifying experience a physician looks forward to.

It is beyond the scope of this book to go into detail about the use of CPAP, but generally speaking, a mask or nasal pillow is firmly adjusted to the face. Tubing attaches the mask to the machine, which forces pressurized air through the tubing to keep airways open during sleep. By keeping the airways open and preventing their collapse, oxygen supply to the body and brain is no longer disrupted and sleep is not interrupted. The patient enjoys an uninterrupted night's sleep and feels rested in the morning. There is no doubt that this involves a period of adjustment, but in most cases, the results are worthwhile. As I mentioned previously, the statistics on the problem of sleep apnea are staggering, and the health impact of untreated sleep disorders is extreme.

Medications that may impact sleep—what to avoid (115)

A number of drugs disrupt sleep, while others can cause daytime drowsiness. Your clinician may be able to suggest alternatives.

Medication	Used to treat	Examples	Possible effects on sleep/day-time function
Anti-arrhythmics	Heart rhythm problems	procainamide (Procanbid), quinidine (Cardioquin), disopyramide (Norpace)	Nighttime sleep difficulties, daytime fatigue
Beta blockers	High blood pressure, heart rhythm problems, angina	atenolol (Tenormin), metoprolol (Lopressor), propranolol (Inderal)	Insomnia, nighttime awakenings, nightmares
Clonidine	High blood pressure; sometimes prescribed off-label for alcohol withdrawal or smoking cessation	clonidine (Catapres)	Daytime drowsiness and fatigue, disrupted REM sleep; less commonly, restlessness, early morning awakening, nightmares
Corticosteroids	Inflammation, asthma	prednisone (Sterapred, others)	Daytime jitters, insomnia
Diuretics	High blood pressure	chlorothiazide (Diuril), chlorthalidone (Hygroton), hydrochlorothiazide (Esidrix, HydroDIURIL, others)	Increased nighttime urination, painful calf cramps during sleep
Medications containing alcohol	Cough, cold, and flu	Coricidin HBP, Nyquil Cough, Theraflu Warming Relief	Suppressed REM sleep, disrupted nighttime sleep

Medications containing caffeine	Decreased alertness	NoDoz, Vivarin, Caffedrine	Wakefulness that may last up to six to seven hours
	Headaches and other pain	Anacin, Excedrin, Midol	
Nicotine replacement products	Smoking	nicotine patches (Nicoderm), gum (Nicorette), nasal spray or inhalers (Nicotrol), and lozenges (Commit)	Insomnia, disturbing dreams
Sedating antihistamines*	Cold and allergy symptoms	diphenhydramine (Benadryl), chlorpheniramine (Chlor-Trimeton)	Drowsiness
	Motion sickness	dimenhydrinate (Dramamine)	
Selective serotonin reuptake inhibitors (SSRIs)	Depression, anxiety	fluoxetine (Prozac), sertraline (Zoloft), paroxetine (Paxil)	Decreased REM sleep, daytime fatigue
Sympathomimetic stimulants	Attention deficit disorder	dextroamphetamine (Dexedrine), methamphetamine (Desoxyn), methylphenidate (Ritalin)	Difficulty falling asleep, decreased REM and non-REM deep sleep
Theophylline	Asthma	theophylline (Slo-bid, Theo-Dur, others)	Wakefulness similar to that caused by caffeine
Thyroid hormone	Hypothyroidism	levothyroxine (Levoxyl, Synthroid, others)	Sleeping difficulties (at higher doses)

*These medications are also found in over-the-counter sleep aids.

Basic Tips for a Good Night's Sleep

Adapted from "When You Can't Sleep: The ABCs of ZZZs," published by the National Sleep Foundation [https://sleepfoundation.org] (116)

- Set a schedule: Go to bed at a set time each night and get up at the same time each morning. Disrupting this schedule may lead to insomnia. "Sleeping in" on weekends also makes it harder to wake up early on Monday morning because it resets your sleep cycles for a later awakening.

- Exercise: Try to exercise twenty to thirty minutes a day. Daily exercise often helps people sleep, although a workout soon before bedtime may interfere with sleep. For maximum benefit, try to get your exercise about five to six hours before going to bed.

- Avoid caffeine, nicotine, and alcohol: Later in the day, stay away from drinks that contain caffeine, which acts as a stimulant and keeps people awake. Sources of caffeine include coffee, chocolate, soft drinks, non-herbal teas, diet drugs and some pain relievers. Smokers tend to sleep very lightly and often wake up in the early morning due to nicotine withdrawal. Despite its mild sedative qualities, alcohol often contributes to poor sleep. Studies have shown that the sedative quality of alcohol is only temporary. Over time, as the body processes alcohol, it begins to stimulate parts of the brain. In many cases this will cause awakenings and sleep problems later in the night.

- Relax before bed: A warm bath, reading, or another relaxing routine can make it easier to fall sleep. You can train yourself to associate certain restful activities with sleep and make them part of your bedtime ritual.

- Sleep until sunlight: If possible, wake up with the sun, or use very bright lights in the morning. Sunlight helps the body's internal biological clock reset itself each day. Sleep experts recommend exposure to an hour of morning sunlight for people who have problems falling asleep.

- Don't lie in bed awake: If you can't get to sleep, don't just lie in bed. Do something else, like reading, watching television or listening to music, until you feel tired. The anxiety of being unable to fall asleep can actually contribute to insomnia.

- Control your room temperature: Maintain a comfortable temperature in the bedroom. Extreme temperatures may disrupt sleep or prevent you from falling asleep.

- See a doctor if your sleeping problem continues: If you have trouble falling asleep night after night, or if you always feel tired the next day, then you may have a sleep disorder and should see a physician. Your primary care physician may be able to help you; if not, you can probably find a sleep specialist at a major hospital near you.

Most sleep disorders can be treated effectively, but you may need to try several solutions or combinations of solutions to get relief. Good sleep hygiene is an important aspect of living GRACEFULLY. My advice is to pay as much attention to your sleep as you would to all of the other elements of the Power of 5 I have referred to in previous chapters. All of the elements are interrelated. In the next chapter I will provide insight and recommendation about how "Sex" is a key element in the power of 5.

Power of 5 Pointers
Chapter 5-Sleep

1. *Animal and human research studies suggest adequate sleep is crucial to a long healthy life.*
2. *There is a strong link between inadequate sleep and most of the inflammatory diseases mentioned in this book such as obesity, diabetes, mood, and cognitive disorders.*
3. *Forty million Americans suffer from sleep disorder and another twenty million have occasional sleep problems. Eighteen million have sleep apnea.*
4. *Sleep apnea can interfere with the management of cognitive disorders, diabetes, congestive heart failure, heartburn and weight gain.*
5. *Develop methods to improve sleep and get seven to eight hours every night. Avoid medications that interfere with sleep.*

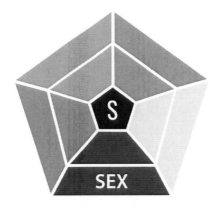

CHAPTER 6

SEX... It is hardly ever just about Sex

ncluding information on sex and human sexuality is essential to the Power of 5 Formula for longevity and remaining youthful. This subject matter deserves focus and attention in our daily lives. Yes, the word "sex" gets people's attention, and we all have heard that "sex sells," but the importance of this topic reinforces my strong desire to educate readers on how we can all AGE GRACEFULLY® through intimacy and companionship.

Here is an example of what I mean when I say that the word sex is a magnet for attention. A few years ago I produced five short YouTube videos to draw attention to myself, my work and to educate viewers about topics relevant to aging. The various subjects included GRACE, Betty White, choosing a retirement community, and sex after eighty. For every single view of any of these videos, my "Sex after 80" exceeded the others by a ratio of twenty to one.

The truth is that sex, intimacy, close physical contact and having meaningful relationships with people is a critical piece of the puzzle to staying healthy and living longer. When we are in the presence of a loved one, we have greater purpose to our life. We eat healthier, exercise more, rest and sleep better, and, hopefully, have less stress. Finding and maintaining intimate connections is also part of what I consider sex. It is not always about the act of sexual intercourse, although that sure adds to the potential pleasure.

As I prepared this section I discovered the research of Robin Dunbar, who has performed a considerable amount of research in this area. The University of Oxford anthropologist and psychologist (then at University College London) was trying to solve the problem of why primates devote so much time and effort to grooming.

In the process of figuring out the solution, he chanced upon a potentially far more intriguing application for his research. It held that the larger the primate's brain, the larger its social circles. By comparing other primates to humans and judging from the size of an average human brain, the number of people the average person could have in her social group was 150. Anything beyond that would be too complicated to handle at optimal processing levels.

For the last twenty-two years, Dunbar has been massaging this data and has produced remarkable insight into social circles of adult humans. The best known, 150, is the number of people we call casual friends—the people, say, you'd invite to a large party. He has broken this down further, and I would direct readers to his research for more information. I have accepted his number, five, as the number of close intimate relationships adults have and have included it in how I visualize the intimate relationships I will discuss in this chapter.

Visualize this concept:

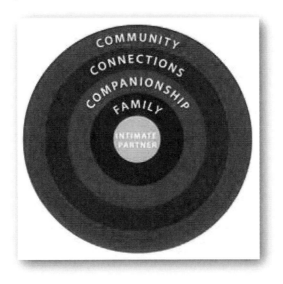

I see five concentric circles moving out from the most intimate level of inti-macy-Sex- followed by Family, then Companionship followed by Connections and finally Community. In this chapter I will describe and give clear examples of each of these relationships (circles) and later will provide methods of developing each.

Intimate Partner

First, I want to address sex from the perspective of a practicing physician and geriatrician.

As a twenty-something adult medical student, I didn't really have a deep understanding of sex and intimacy. My medical school training focused lim-ited attention on the subject. We had a crash course that included desensiti-zation exercises to help us feel more comfortable and less judgmental as we counseled our patients, including older adults, on this subject. Once I started my own practice, I had to be able to jump right in and talk about issues regard-ing sex as if I was an expert, just like Dr. Ruth Westheimer. This approach con-sumed a lot of energy on my part. Over time, I became better at interacting with my patients, allowing them to feel comfortable about confiding in me about intimacy in their lives.

Our views on human sexuality, especially in the U.S., are heavily influenced by the media. If people lived their lives like the characters in some movies I have seen, they would be in and out of bed many times a week and possibly with multiple partners. As I have interacted with patients in my practice and explored the literature, I have concluded that we are more tame than we are portrayed in the movies. Younger adults do have more time, energy, and curi-osity and do have more active sex lives than older adults, but I have discovered there is a natural evolution. After an initial infatuation in a relationship, sexual activity declines. When the relationship matures and jobs and family take a higher precedence, sexual activity often declines further.

Let me introduce my patients Amanda and Bill. They knew each other in high school but started dating only when he joined the police force and she began her job as a graphic designer. After a two-year courtship, they married. As they tell me, they had a very active sex life, becom-ing intimate two or three times a week. Once she became pregnant, things changed dramatically. They remained in love, but sex took a back seat while they were raising children. Additionally, one of their children had special needs, a circumstance that added emotional and physical drains on the energy resources, curtailing periods of intimacy. That is not to say they didn't have sex, but it was less frequent, spontaneous, and shorter in duration. To hear Amanda tell it, "We were still in love but did not have much time to express it." Bill would tell me that working on the police force had its disadvantages as well. "Some weeks I had to work stakeouts at night and did not have the time or energy to connect with Amanda."

Since they have remained healthy patients of mine, I have had the good fortune to check in on them from time to time. Their children got older and they indicated they had more time, energy and opportunity to be intimate with each other. Once their youngest was off to college, they resumed a more active sex life, and each felt more connected to the other.

Amanda and Bill have been very fortunate that they were able to rekindle the intimate sexual relationship they had when they were younger. Not all couples are so fortunate.

In our hectic lives, it would be easy to lose the spark that you and your mate/partner shared when you were younger. Maintaining a date night or some other activity that allows you to keep the flame burning can be crucial to sustaining intimacy in your fifties and later life. As we see in the studies reported by reputable research centers, intimacy in the older adult can be directly related to what occurred in all the years prior.

Sexuality in later life

According to the sexual research group The Kinsey Institute, there is no age limit on sexuality and sexual activity. While the frequency or ability to perform sexually will generally decline modestly as seniors experience the normal physiological changes that accompany aging, reports show that the majority of men and women between the ages of fifty and eighty are still enthusiastic about sex and intimacy. One such example is my patient Glenda, whom I have treated for many years.

Over the years I have had many encounters with patients like seventy-four-year-old Glenda. Our conversation during an office visit a few years ago revolved around the medications she was taking and whether or not she felt they would continue to be effective for her. When I asked her about her sleep patterns, she indicated that some nights her sleep was disrupted and she had a difficult time getting back to sleep. As I considered that she might have symptoms of sleep apnea, I asked if she would consent to being tested. When she hesitated to respond I indicated that if I discovered she had sleep apnea she could be fitted for a mask to wear in bed while sleeping. In an effort to put her at ease and break the tension, I said with tongue in cheek, "Since you don't have sex any more it won't be a hindrance to that activity."

She reacted to this remark with a look that revealed I was dead wrong.

Unlike many other seventy-four-year-olds, she had not given up sexual activity. Furthermore, she informed me she had no intention of stopping because of a sleep apnea diagnosis. Glenda went on to describe the wonderful relationship with her adoring husband and her very active, intimate relationship with him.

I did let her know I was just teasing her, not wanting to make her feel uncomfortable by assuming that she was active when she might not have been. Glenda indicated that she and many of her similarly aged friends remain sexually active with their spouses and discussed the subject frequently. She further explained that she and her husband were best friends and enjoyed the time they spent together in their retirement. They shared many of the same interests and loved to travel together.

In addition to the sexually intimate relationship Glenda had with her husband, she had many other intimate non-sexual relationships with female friends. She especially bonded with the women she attended exercise class with, looking forward to their weekly lunch together. She had one friend in particular who was also a patient of mine. They were separated in age by nearly twenty years, but had a special fondness for each other, almost like mother and daughter. "I live for the connections I have with my close friends. These relationships keep me young at heart and connected," Glenda told me.

I will return to these types of connections and community later in this chapter.

What is evident to me is that the phenomenon of "use it or lose it" holds true in the story about Glenda and her husband. Human sexuality thrives on a repetitive process that includes an enhanced flow of blood to sexual organs. This blood flow further enhances the long-term viability of the sexual organs. When adults stay interested, remain healthy, limit prescription and non-prescription medications and have a committed partner with similar ideals, they can have satisfying sex for as long as they live.

A Duke University study shows that some twenty percent of people over sixty-five have sex lives that are better than ever before. And although not everyone wants or needs an active sex life, many people continue to be sexual all their lives. (117)

Dr. Walter Bortz, past president of the American Geriatrics Society and professor at Stanford Medical School, was quoted as saying, "There's strong data all over: it's a matter of survival that people that have sex live longer. Married people live longer. People need people. The more intimate the connection, the more powerful the effects."

Another example of the urge to forge a connection is illustrated in my patient Anthony.

Anthony had been a typical patient in my practice for many years. His ailing wife had severe COPD and was treated exclusively by her lung specialist. In our discussions, he reported that he enjoyed an active sex life with his wife until her condition deteriorated, when all intimacy in their relationship ended. He was a devoted husband and offered no complaints, just the observation of his loss. He did continue to provide love and support to his wife through her long illness, until the moment of her death.

He and I would speak often of the prolonged suffering his wife had with her illness. "She would have done the same for me if the tables were turned," he told me many times.

After her death, I provided Anthony with the comfort I believe a caring physician should offer and he opened up a great deal about their life together. "I was a military man, you know, and I worked up to the rank of colonel. I was fortunate to be stationed with my wife and kids all over the world. I really liked it when I was stationed in Germany. We had lots of opportunities to travel, and we enjoyed each other's company and had a wonderful sex life. I was good to her and she was good to me. I will really miss that," he confessed one day.

In keeping with his love of international travel he told me about an Elderhostel trip he took to Spain. "I had a real annoying roommate on the trip. He snored like an army tank and I had to get out of the room for long stretches of time." Early in the trip, while escaping his army tank, he met a woman who suffered a similar fate: her roommate had a horrible cough and made loud wheezing sounds for hours. They shared a drink in the lounge and it became a regular routine for them on the trip. It turned out that they lived less than twenty miles from one another and began dating soon after their return home. Anthony was sixty-six when they met and Estelle was sixty. What was so remarkable about their coupleship was that he had been married from age nineteen, but she had never married. She had made a commitment to her parents that she would take care of them until they died. They lived into their late eighties before she was released from her personal commitment.

I have always marveled about the relationship they developed—he who had been married to the same woman for forty years and she who had never had an intimate relationship. What I did learn was that based on her relationship with her parents, she was a caring, devoted woman willing to make many sacrifices. Anthony and Estelle were married. I had the good fortune to have a solid enough relationship with Anthony, and support for him in the early years of his marriage especially, that I was able to inquire if they had any problems with intimacy in light of the fact that Estelle had never been married.

"We have a great love life, Doc. She had a good idea of what to do from the get go and was very amenable to discussing what I could do to enhance her satisfaction and her mine." I managed his care for the subsequent twenty happy years of his life.

Strange as it may seem, older people may encounter an obstacle they hadn't expected: their adult children, who may be less than pleased to see their aging parents as sexual beings. This can be especially true when a parent seeks a new intimate connection after losing a partner to death or divorce.

Judgmental attitudes prevent many older people from moving in with each other or even having their partner over. This type of attitude can create obstacles for many seniors who want to be sexually active.

Seniors hooking up may well lose some of its taboo status, however, as the baby boom generation enters its later years. With their increased numbers and a marked increase in life expectancy, older adults are now the fastest-growing segment of the U.S. population. According to the U.S. Census Bureau in 2000, one out of ten Americans was sixty-five years or older. By the year 2030, it is estimated that one in every five Americans will be sixty-five or over. (118)

The next patient, Mary, turned out to be a good example of seniors hooking up late in life.

Falling in love at any age

Mary is an even older patient who demonstrated you are never too old for romance.

Mary is a fairly new patient in my practice although I have taken care of many other members of her extended family. Her husband, George, had become a patient after his physician retired. I had just a short time to treat him before he died.

Mary told me they had an active sex life until he became a diabetic and had prostate cancer. These health issues eventually curtailed their sexual activity but did not stop either of them from becoming intimate in other ways, such as having close physical contact frequently during the day. After George died, Mary was shaken, her spirit was negatively affected, and she became withdrawn and depressed. Months later, on a follow-up visit, she mentioned that an old acquaintance from childhood had attended her husband's funeral. He had asked her to have lunch when things settled down and when she was ready. Mary and I discussed his offer, and on many occasions Mary told me that she was just too sad and missed George so much she couldn't think of having lunch with anyone, let alone an old man who lived forty miles away.

At the next visit, Mary indicated she had lunch with the old acquaintance we had spoken about. She described the encounter as "nice and cordial," indicating she might visit him in a few weeks.

Mary came to her next office visit as excited as any eighty-six-year-old love-struck person I have ever seen. She behaved with the same kind of infatuation that I have seen in twenty- and thirty-year olds who just couldn't wait for their next visit together. As she told me, "It did not take long to feel comfortable with him, and before we knew it our clothes were off. You know, doctor, you never know how long you're going to live and you can't waste any time. Sex keeps a person active and alive."

Her experience supports my observations and those of many experts that patterns of sexuality can be set earlier in life. In addition, the biological changes associated with aging are less pronounced and sexuality is less affected if sexual activity is constant throughout life. With less time to devote to family, seniors can devote more time and energy to improving their love lives. Some seniors may be forced to give up strenuous sports, whereas sex is a physical pleasure many older people readily enjoy.

According to a survey by AARP, the clear majority of men and women aged forty-five and up say that a satisfying sexual relationship is important to their quality of life. Among those forty-five to fifty-nine with sexual partners, some fifty-six percent said they had sexual intercourse once a week or more. Among sixty- to seventy-year-olds with partners, forty-six percent of men and thirty-eight percent of women have sex at least once a week, as did thirty-four percent of those seventy or older. (119)

Similar findings emerged in a survey conducted by the National Council on Aging (NCOA). The study, reported by multiple news outlets in 1998, found that nearly half of all Americans age sixty or over have sex at least once a month and that nearly half also wanted to have sex more frequently. Another finding: people find their mates more physically attractive over time. (120) I did find it interesting that the study was, in fact, partially financed by an unrestricted grant from Pfizer Inc., the producers of the anti-impotence drug Viagra.

The Partner Gap

The physical changes that occur with age can give older people a chance to revitalize their lovemaking by focusing more on intimacy and closeness instead of sex alone. Often less preoccupied with performance, they can express their affection and closeness in other ways, such as cuddling, kissing and stroking.

But among older women who are widowed, divorced or single, finding a partner can be difficult. According to several reports, women make up the majority of the elderly without partners. The reasons: women live longer than men, and healthy older men tend to pair up with younger women. Older women are also judged by society as less attractive than their male counterparts, a double standard that women's groups have long decried.

This "partner gap" greatly inhibits women's social and sexual activity as they reach their senior years. In the AARP study, only thirty-two percent of women seventy or older have partners, compared with fifty-nine percent of men in the same age group. In the NCOA study, older men are more likely than older women to be married and have sex partners.

Dr. Ruth Westheimer has written extensively on the subject of sex. (121) As it relates to this subject she has broken her thoughts down in the following way. We must be aware of the physical changes we go through as well as those of the opposite sex. Without an understanding of the changes our bodies go through as we age, we are destined for disappointment and confusion. The fact is that as we age our ability to achieve the same kinds of pleasure in the same way has changed. It is also clear that for successful intimacy to occur we must evaluate both our physical and emotional fitness. A balance of a healthy body and mind is essential to enjoying the intimacy one desires. Dr. Ruth would remind us to spice up our love life, including games, toys and erotica—if these are things one is comfortable with are not offensive to the partner.

Those who are trying to find a partner have to consider that how you present yourself and how prepared you are for meeting someone are of upmost importance. It is important to attend the types of activities that will put you in places where you will have opportunities to meet someone. One has to decide whether to go alone to an event or go with a friend for support. When looking, it is more effective if you "tell the world you are looking." Avoid being too picky. Be honest. If you expect someone to be honest with you, start from that point and always be honest in your interactions. It can become very uncomfortable if you have to disclose some disingenuous piece of information once a relationship has picked up steam.

Returning to the concepts postulated by Robin Dunbar, I regard the following five types of connections as easily identifiable in our lives and worth considering as we give our lives perspective.

Family—close bonds, unconditional love and support

In the graphic that opens this chapter, Family forms the next level of intimacy. Even though we don't choose our families, we cannot help sharing genetic material and, if all goes well, we will have connections for life. One would hope that when all is said and done, it is a lasting connection we can count on if all others fail. Many people find such love and sustenance in these relationships.

One such example is that of Stephanie and her sister Ellen. These two of the four siblings in their family have remained the most connected. Much of it has to do with the eighteen-month age difference and shared experiences when they were growing up. As they matured they remained confidants, supporting each other through their many accomplishments and challenges. When parents or the other siblings in the family became ill or suffered one setback, as a team they were involved and supportive as if they were tending to each other. Stephanie, in particular, due to her work schedule, would drop whatever she was doing to attend to a family member's needs. Regardless of geographic separation and the medical ailments each has had to address, they have maintained the "close, loving, intimate relationship" that with luck and effort can be shared by siblings in a family.

The bonds of family are magical. While they might survive without much attention, working to maintain the relationship fosters and enables them to thrive.

Companionship—close intimate friends

As we work out from the center of this intimacy schematic, I would identify the next as Companionship—those five close relationships that Robin Dunbar describes. Most people could identify five individuals in their lives at any one time who could fit the bill as those truly intimate people. These are the friends you could call on at a moment's notice; they know you so well that they know how you think and can help you in a time of paralysis. **These are intense relationships, I suspect, between individuals of the same sex but are as strong and lasting as those between a husband and wife.**

> One such relationship I have observed is between Peggy Sue and Janet. They met in religious school when they were just eight years old. They lost contact during high school, as many children do, but reconnected in college. They have been like sisters to each other ever since. They have nurtured each other through the challenges of marriage, divorce, work, hardships with family, and health crises. Each has dropped whatever she was doing at the time to provide immediate support when needed. They speak on the phone many times a week and are aware of the intimate details of each other's lives. There is never a question whether either person will be available. It is a 24/7 unconditional love and support.

Connections—book club members, mahjong groups, golf buddies, fraternity brothers or sorority sisters, co-workers

The next ring in my schematic is what I identify as Connections. Most of us can recognize this group of ten to thirty friends. It is those we might have over for dinner, hang out with in book clubs or mahjong groups. For men it might be guys we play golf, cards or poker with, and it can even include co-workers. Couples do this in the form of bridge partners, bowling teams, or even mixed doubles tennis and golf groups.

What might have started out as a group of individuals with a common purpose, if held together long enough often evolves into a group of highly supportive adults who can have a surprising influence in times of need for companionship. I am always delighted to hear about how a patient's group of friends rallies to his or her side when support of one sort or another is needed.

In my professional experience, I have seen this among a group of retired Salvation Army officers. In their professional lives they worked with each other in different locations toward a common goal, leading their organization. In retirement they became a family. This tight-knit group of friends went to church together, had dinner after church and supported each other in their daily lives. Many of the men played golf together, even as they recognizing their performance was terrible. Since most were retired in Florida, their imme-diate family was out of state, further encouraging this supportive network to develop and strengthen.

Another such example is that of my wife and her friend Veronica.

Veronica is a lovely, caring woman and seemed to always be there in time of need for friends in her book club. As Veronica and her husband neared retirement, they would spend more and more time in another state. During one of the blocks of time when they were in town we heard about an injury her son had sustained in a motor vehicle accident. It did not take long for the troops to mobilize. They provided emo-tional support, were at Veronica's side and provided meals for her so she would not have to be preoccupied with feeding herself and her husband. It was easy for this group of friends to provide this type of support as they too had become like sisters to each other through the bonding of their activities in their book club.

The sense of intimacy in this type of relationship is special. It may not be sex, but it is very close and special.

Community—church and civic group, boards

This next and last ring in my schematic is the most outer one that I will address. It represents our relations in our Community. These are the people we see regularly in our community. The community might be a large corporation, reli-gious organization, civic organization or community board. While I have had relationships myself in each of the circles mentioned in this chapter, I have not included myself in any of the stories until now.

Shortly after settling into my community I was invited to serve on the board of Jewish Family Services. At the time I was not certain exactly what this board did, and since I was no more than thirty-five years old, I had no previous experience as a board member. I figured I would give it a try. It was really an easy decision, as I had always wanted to do some type of volunteering in my community. I would soon learn the many facets of the organization and the breadth of other volunteers serving actively on the board.

The energy of the other board members amazed me, and so did the impact the organization had on the individuals it served. A byproduct of my participation was my association with many different energetic and professionally successful individuals with whom I formed bonds. Many served as role models for me in many ways; they were people I looked up to.

I have developed bonds over the years I have been on this community board that have broadened my view of the world and connected me to people I would never have met, allowing me to add to the circle of relationships that have strengthened my life.

Conclusion

As you can see from the concentric circles in my schematic view, sex and intimacy is for everyone, regardless of class, gender, or age. All individuals have to find where they fit within the concentric circles and recognize their area of sex/intimacy. If you are human, the closeness that comes from interaction with others and the warm feelings derived from connections and support are an important component of living and growing older GRACEfully.

In our society it's true that seniors more frequently experience the loss of a loved one, partners or close friends. But these last chapters of life can be fulfilling. Those who age GRACEfully benefit from close relationships with others. They enhance their lives from lessons learned. Regardless of age, very satisfying relationships, both old and new, remain possible.

S is for Sex— Formula
The Importance of Intimacy, Companionship and Connection

In addition to meeting certain human biological needs, the emotional bond that sex promotes is very special. We cannot stand alone. We need real connections to others in our universe. The results of that relationship and those with our immediate family are lifetime connections. They have special importance.

Forging and maintaining lifelong friendships is another way to ensure the companionship and connections that provide support and comfort when family is neither accessible nor available. We begin many of these relationships in childhood. They develop more deeply and powerfully as we progress through our years in school and starting out in the world afterward.

As we move through life, developing these types of relationships becomes more difficult. Looking for and finding them can be a challenge, so we have to be more intentional about making friends and acquaintances. We need to put ourselves out there at our place of work or join groups (such as churches and synagogues, or other affinity groups) to meet people who share common interests. Another way is to develop a hobby or join a group where you can meet people. Mahjong or bridge groups and golf or bowling leagues are among some very accessible options. Joining a club that travels, or the Red Hat Society, or a singing group like the Sweet Adelines could provide opportunities to flaunt your talent and, at the same time, meet like-minded people. Taking a class at a local college or adult education program, or a local photography class may put you in contact with others who share common interests as well.

If it is not people you need, consider adopting a pet. Animals are capable of providing considerable companionship. Believe it or not, at the very least, a pet will give you something to talk about when you are in social situations, where new relationships can be forged as well. Taking your dog to a dog park is an excellent way to interact with other people who share common interests and concerns.

It may sound banal, but invite friends over for dinner. My wife and I have established a great way to get together with our existing friends and introduce them to others. We've developed a list of forty or fifty of the favorite people in our lives and invite them to join us for dinner once a month on a Friday night. We think it's a great way to start the weekend off right. We use an online software program called "Doodle," where the guest RSVPs without knowing who else would be attending that night. We limit each dinner to twelve guests. When they arrive, they are surprised to see who else is in attendance. We all have a great night, the conversation is always different and stimulating, and everyone compliments me on my grandmother's chicken soup recipe and on the delicious healthy meals my wife, Melissa, has prepared.

Initiation of relationships and online dating

One hundred and fifty years ago there was no such thing as dating. In most societies, marriages were arranged. This tradition still exists in some cultures in this world. It is likely that my paternal grandparents were brought together by a matchmaker in their village in Poland during the late 1800s. Fifty years later my parents were set up on a blind date and met at a skating rink in Manhattan with very little fanfare. After a short courtship they married, just like millions of other post-World War II Americans.

Circumstances are very different in this century. With the advent of superhighways, transcontinental airline travel, and a global economy; people meet, relationships develop, and marriages occur between people of all nationalities. With these changes of the last 150 years, dating patterns have changed as well. It used to be that people had to be introduced or meet in a bar. Nowadays young people either meet in their college dormitory or dating channels such as "It's about Lunch," "Meet Up" socials or internet sites (more about that later). But what about mature adults in their forties, fifties and all the way up to their eighties and nineties? What do they do? Are they still interested in dating, relationships, and intimacy? How do they go about finding one another?

In considering their options, I want to revisit a survey conducted by the National Council on Aging (NCOA) that I mentioned earlier in this chapter. The study found that nearly half of all Americans age sixty or over have sex at least once a month and that nearly half also wanted to have sex more frequently. Interpreting this data confirms what I have been stressing throughout this chapter about the need and desire of adults of all ages to maintain intimate relationships. Currently, adults of all ages would use whatever means possible to meet individuals for that purpose. For this age group, online dating has become a very popular method of meeting new people and initiating a warm and possibly intimate relationship.

There are many online dating services offering either free or paid memberships. One needs to do just a little bit of homework or surfing the internet to find one that would help discover that special someone. Match.com is the largest, and others, like Plenty of Fish and eHarmony are well-known sites. Then there are boutique sites that target any special need you could think of. There are sites such as JDate (Jewish dating), Christian Mingle, GayDate, Tinder, and sites for people with special interests like FitSingles for fitness buffs.

Searching for companionship and love has become really easy. Anyone with knowledge of internet basics and an internet connection can join one of these sites.

If this is an avenue you wish to travel, here are some thoughts to consider as you pursue online dating.

Make sure you're ready: When a relationship ends either through divorce or death of a spouse or companion, it's worthwhile to take an appropriate period of time to be certain you're ready to share yourself with another person. Make sure that you're mentally healthy, as it is a daunting task to find someone well-suited for you. You want to make certain that you are no longer angry or grieving or sad or in the wrong place to enter a relationship. If you're not ready, seek counseling from friends, family or a therapist.

Preparation is important: Make sure you investigate and find the right dating service for you. You may want to try more than one site.

Ask for help: this is where experienced friends come in—to help select appropriate photos and develop a profile. During my research for this section, I discovered that there are professional coaches who help potential daters write catchy prose to generate attention. Choosing the right words to use in a profile is important. I recommend avoiding the use of the same expressions everyone else uses (like "I enjoy romantic walks on the beach at sunset"). Who doesn't enjoy that?

Be open to adventure: avoid using negative words or expressions that would put limitations on yourself. If you set your standard or your date's standards too high you will never get a date (like saying you are interested only in doctors with degrees from Harvard).

Safety: Safety is always my number-one rule as a physician. It applies here. Avoid initiating contact even by phone until you feel comfortable. Avoid using a home phone that could be linked to your home address. When setting up a meeting, do so in a public place. Meeting for coffee is a well-accepted first date.

Drive yourself to and from the date. Park your car in a non-secluded, well-lit spot. Walk by yourself to your car. Do not take any undue risks.

Be patient: You will have to spend time and review a lot of pictures and profiles to select ones you might want to reach out to. Online dating is difficult; don't expect to fall in love immediately.

Be prepared for the challenge: I like the expression "no expectations, no disappointments." If it is meant to be, it will happen.

Find enjoyment in the process: Just as I recommended in the section about exercise, make it an enjoyable process, not torture.

Medications to enhance intimacy:

Whether you have found that new relationship and you plan to take it to the next level or if your relationship has spanned decades, one must consider the possibility of the physical challenges associated with being intimate. Before getting into specifics, you may recall that I discovered that the NCOA survey I referred to in the previous section was conveniently sponsored by Pfizer, the company that manufactures and markets the first in a new line of medication to come to market for erectile dysfunction. As a major publicly traded pharmaceutical company, Pfizer had a responsibility to its shareholders to do its due diligence to be certain that there would be demand for its novel product. The results of the survey and the track record for sales of Viagra have demonstrated a strong and growing interest in medication to help enhance intimacy between partners.

It is well known that Viagra and its competitors, Cialis and Levitra have been enormously successful and popular, suggesting a strong desire—at least among men—to remain sexually active. I have had men into their nineties ask for a prescription for the "blue pill"; and they were not shy about asking.

Some studies also suggest that the supplement ginkgo biloba, which increases circulation, can help treat impotence, but others show no such effect. In my career I have not heard of any of my patients having success with this product. Men should always check with their doctors before taking it. Among other things, ginkgo can interact with anticoagulants, thereby creating additional problems.

Despite the potential benefits of prescription medication, studies show that only a fraction of the individuals who could be treated for sexual problems actually seek medical help. That's unfortunate because even serious medical conditions need not prevent elders from having a satisfying intimacy and sexual relations. Men (even with their partner) should see a physician if they've lost interest in sex or are having sexual difficulties. Some sedatives, most antidepressants, excessive alcohol, and some prescription drugs have side effects that interfere with erections and sex. Physicians can help adjust medication or set guidelines on alcohol intake. Illnesses, disabilities, and surgeries can also affect sexuality, but in general, even disease need not interfere with sexual expression.

Women are a different story, and I am prepared to include only a few remarks on the subject. Men and women are different when it comes to intimacy. Women want at least a little romance and foreplay. If they don't get any, it is difficult for them to become aroused or interested. There has been no effective medication for women that promotes prompt arousal as Viagra does for men. For women the diminished interest is partly hormonal, partly societal norm, and partly attitude related to the relationship with the companion. What it comes down to is that the man is the medication; the key ingredient to the woman's ignition, not a pill that has to be swallowed.

I will address this later in this chapter but for now I will provide four things to think about as the male replacement for Viagra. **Pay attention** to your partner; compliment her appearance—her hair, smile, clothing. **Listen to her and remember** what she enjoys and finds stimulating both emotionally and physically. **Do those things** to her that she tells you she enjoys as often as you can. **Be the gentleman** she wishes to have. Chivalry is not dead.

Examples of things to do may include: make it a habit to open the car door for her getting into and out of the car; plan special date nights; take control of situations so she can appreciate the powerful and caring man you are. The message to men here is clear; if he wants to share intimacy with his woman, this is the prescription/pill.

Additionally, one of the most important factors is keeping lines of communication open with your companion about what works and how to make the intimate moments enjoyable for both participants.

Managing physical limitations:

As a practicing physician I have discussed physical limitation periodically with my patients and I have often been frustrated. Most physicians and I really do not have the expertise or the time during any regular office visit to address these critical patient concerns. Many of the issues relate to the conditions addressed in the four previous chapters in the book; **stress, sweets, sweat and sleep**. Individuals who are **stressed,** depressed or taking medication to address these issues have problems with libido and energy to perform. Overdoing it with **Sweets** contributes to diabetes and cardiovascular diseases, and can affect vascular supply to sex organs and diminish performance. **Sweat**, or lack of exercise and physical activity, correlates to diminished testosterone and libido with diminished interest and performance. Finally those who suffer from a **sleep** disorder cannot find the energy or interest to initiate intimacy.

Obesity presents its own set of challenges—both from the diminished testosterone and self-esteem and from limits related to size. Those patients with orthopedic conditions such as arthritic hips, knees, or spines find it difficult and painful to make the physical connections. Patients with chronic lung disease have problems with endurance and libido.

There is no easy access to manuals that could help overcome different medical conditions. The guidance I offer is similar to what I read in Dr. Ruth Westheimer's work. She advises that "you have to take it slow and experiment with your partner to find what works" and "don't be bashful or you might miss out on pleasurable experiences."

I anticipate doing further research on this subject and publishing a book to address this subject in greater detail.

Finally, be imaginative. Look for opportunities to meet with existing friends or to establish new friendships that can last a lifetime. This, like all the other lifestyle modifications I'm suggesting in this book, requires intention.

The Power of 5 essential components to develop and maintain intimacy and relationships

Here are five elements that can be helpful in leading to the success of an intimate relationship. They can also be utilized in many other relationships such as at work, on an athletic team or with any other individuals you encounter in life.

Be present, listen, and pay attention

In order for any relationship to even start, you must be present. "You will never get a second date with the person of your dreams if you don't make it to the first one," as one of my more astute patients reminded me. Many people are so frightened of rejection that fear holds them back from even taking the first few steps needed to start a relationship. To get started, you need to take a deep breath and take the plunge. This holds true even more so within a committed relationship, where you must remain present and attentive to your partner.

Once the flames of a relationship have blazed up, it is important to remain in the moment and to use your skill as a listener. The person to whom you are relating expects you to pay attention to every word. As you pay attention, you must also remember and be prepared to recall what you have heard. As I have interviewed many of the patients in my practice who have had successful relationships, they have recited the same phrase over and over: "In order for things to work in my marriage, Doc, I have learned that we must pay attention and listen to each other."

Know your partner

The next element in a successful relationship is the importance of knowing your partner. Whether the relationship has been of short or long duration, the partners have an appropriate expectation that their mate "knows them."

One surefire way to the doghouse is to buy a wife tickets to a hockey game when she continually expresses her desire for tickets to the opera. I recognize that is a tall order for this spouse, but his opportunity to enhance the level of intimacy in his relationship is to go out for a nice dinner and take his wife to the opera. Spouses like the idea that their companion pays attention to the small stuff. Knowing the right perfume to buy or how she likes her coffee is a real turn-on for a companion.

Have patience and relax

Being patient with one another and accepting differences are critical features in healthy relationships. Accepting the things we cannot change in our companion enables us to have considerable freedom in the relationship. Critical to its success is also a matter of being calm. We need to be able to step back from all of the chaos and patiently focus on our partner. Taking time away from our busy work commitments, on either short or long vacations, can ease the tensions in our lives.

In addition and as I mentioned in other parts of the book, learning techniques to relax together can be very helpful. Attending a yoga class or learning how to meditate together will go a long way to solidify a relationship. I remember the husband and wife patients of mine many years ago going through a difficult time both with regard to their health and in the relationship. One day they arrived at my office glowing and holding hands. I asked them, "What have you done to overcome some of the stress and turmoil of the relationship?"

As they held hands and looked into each other's eyes, they told me, "We just started doing tai chi and it has made a remarkable difference in how we feel personally about one another in our relationship."

Have a sense of humor and be adventurous

When I read about successful marriages and in our relationships and what people say about their own successes, they frequently point out that they love their companion's sense of humor. They love the fact that they are able to let down their hair and laugh and joke with each other (of course in a respectful way). Laughter brings out the best in us, causes the release of endorphins and other neurotransmitters, and makes us happy and peaceful in our relationship. For the most part, happy couples enjoy being surprised. After being together for many years, some folks have a tendency to get into a rut, doing the same thing over and over. It gets boring for one or both of the people in the relationship. Being able to spice things up and do adventurous things injects new excitement. Adventure also releases endorphins and happy hormones. When we venture out on skinny branches, this excitement gets our blood flowing. It provides memorable experiences that further solidify the bond in our relationship.

Sometimes those adventurous experiences have to be well planned and thus lack spontaneity, but that's okay. In other situations complete spontaneity can be low maintenance and provides the same level of excitement and further bonding.

Get help to get better

Not all relationships are easy and smooth. Some relationships hit rocky points and need professional counseling. Other relationships do great for a while but fall into difficulties. The people involved in the relationship can benefit from counseling to make them able to handle the difficulties even better. Guidance comes in many shapes and sizes.

Some relationship problems are more deeply rooted; others might be for more focused problems such as difficulty with sexuality and intimacy. Whether you are early in your relationship or in it for fifty years, it is never too early and never too late to ask for help to make it work better.

One such couple, Robert and Kathy, was in the midst of raising their children when they started to struggle in their relationship. Kathy was a deeply religious woman committed to attending church and following the lessons of the Bible. Robert had been consuming more alcohol and began to use cocaine. He felt unappreciated as the provider for the family as all of Kathy's attention was directed toward her children or her church. As they drifted further apart and experienced financial difficulties, Robert started to commit petty crimes and deal in the drug trade. All came crashing down when he was arrested and convicted for his crimes and went to prison. Kathy utilized her connections in her church to find ways of forgiving Robert for his behavior. While in prison Robert focused his energy on eliminating drugs and alcohol from his system and discovering ways to make amends to his wife. Robert and Kathy turned to their church and received the counseling they needed. They continue to have a committed affiliation with their church and with each other. Each credits the counseling they received during their journey as the glue that holds them together today.

As I conclude this section on Sex and Intimacy, I hope it has become clear that the **Power of 5** is a tightly intertwined group of elements that lead to better health, well-being, and longevity. Sex and intimacy might even be the emotional glue that holds the **Power of 5** together. The four other elements are individual activities, but sex and intimacy involves a partner and that in itself sets it apart. When we involve another individual in our lives it not only enhances happiness but it provides an extra incentive to be healthier and live longer.

That is what the **Power of 5** is really about.

The Power of 5 is all about my best advice for living life well for as long as possible. Much of the preventable disease in our world has to do with inflammation. The Power of 5 Formula addresses the root causes of inflamma-tion. **All of the elements of the Power of 5 Formula are modifiable by you!**

I have provided you with a great deal of background and context as well as practical information and strategies for improving those aspects of health and well-being.

I exposed **sweets** as the real villain in our food choices and what we can do to eliminate and replace it. As individuals and as a society we must recognize this is modifiable and a major contributor to illness and premature death.

I revealed **stress** as a subtle but dangerous element that is pervasive in our society and contributes to inflammation and disease as well as to unhappiness. I have given clear and concise methods to help modify stress.

I have highlighted how **sweat** and exercise can reduce inflammation and reduce risk for developing most of the disease I see every day. I have provided the **Power of 5** activities/exercises that can be chosen or mixed and matched and easily implemented into your own **Power of 5** plans.

I have demonstrated the dangers of inadequate quality and duration of **sleep**. Without this vital process our brains and body do not function properly. This situation can ultimately lead to inflammation and cognitive decline. I have provided several recipes for getting a better night's sleep and encouragement to consult with a physician if your sleep is inadequate.

In the final section of part one of this book I have introduced the concept that **Sex** and intimacy are vital to our health and longevity. I know that using the glue of intimacy will lead to more fulfilling relationship, greater happiness, and greater longevity.

Part 2 of this book is about adopting the eating portion of the lifestyle changes I have recommended throughout this book. I will provide clear guidance about what to eat, in what proportion of each meal and what your table setting should look like. I will make it easy to make the changes and experience them at home as well as those occasions when you eat away from home.

Good luck and here's to a long and healthy life!

Power of 5 Pointers
Chapter 6-Sex

1. *The truth is that sex, intimacy, close physical contact and meaningful relationships with people is a critical piece of the puzzle to stay healthy and live longer.*
2. *I see four concentric circles moving out from the most intimate level of intimacy—Sex, followed by Family, then Companionship, followed by Connections and, finally, Community.*
3. *According to a survey by AARP, the clear majority of men and women aged forty-five and up say that a satisfying sexual relationship is important to their quality of life.*
4. *Here are five elements that can be helpful in leading to the success of an intimate relationship:*
    a. *Be present, listen, and pay attention.*
    b. *Know your partner.*
    c. *Have patience and relax.*
    d. *Have a sense of humor and be adventurous.*
    e. *Get help to get better.*
5. *Sex and intimacy might even be the emotional glue that holds the Power of 5 together.*

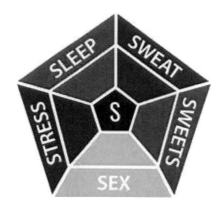

Part II: Putting Healthy Eating into Practice

Menus/Recipes for Longevity Lifestyle

The evidence presented in the first part of this book explores the science behind poor food choices and how this lifestyle impacts bodily functions. This information serves as the motivation for making concrete adjustments or even complete changes. This second part will provide the actionable steps by providing heart-friendly recipes to kick-start your journey to a better, healthier life. It is designed to promote better health and prevent disease by improving choices of what is eaten.

The Power of 5 Formula is all about taking back power and responsibility for the quality of your life, longevity and remaining youthful. My recommendations are geared not only toward weight loss, but to a weight loss as a natural and likely byproduct of one's lifestyle change.

What you will find is an easy to follow eating style similar to that of people who live in what is considered the Mediterranean region of the globe. I believe this eating style is the healthiest, easiest, most affordable, portable, and flexible that I know. The recommended foods are packed with fresh fruits and vegetables, which are plentiful and readily available in most developed countries. There are certain vegetables such as potatoes and other root vegetables that are high in starchy carbohydrates, that I consider taboo. Fruits with high concentrations of sugar should also be eliminated.

Successful adaptation to the Power of 5 eating lifestyle will be easier if you follow specific guidelines. I have provided illustrations of a plate and table settings for each meal with the proper percentage of each food category. I have done as much as I can to keep things simple so they may be easily adapted and applied every day to every meal. All the recipes have been concocted, tasted and adjusted in our very own "**Power of 5 Test Kitchen,**" as my wife and I refer to our culinary laboratory.

My goal was to eliminate a lot of thinking. In the ancient days when our ancestors roamed around the Mediterranean region, not a lot of thinking went into their meal choices. My watchwords are "simple" and "portable," so that when you choose to eat food away from home, you will find it easy to make the conversion.

You will notice no bread (or butter/oil for the bread) on my table setting. Why? Because this type of carbohydrates is not part of the Power of 5 lifestyle.

General Rules:
    Eat all meals on small plates.
    Follow the list of unlimited vegetables.
    Drink a non-caloric beverage with each meal.

Breakfast

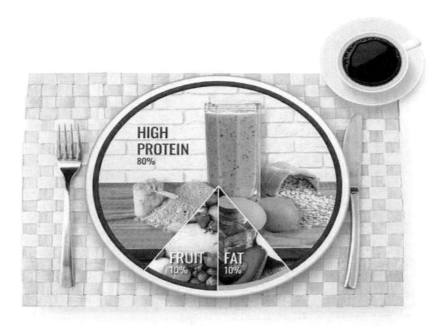

75-80% egg recipe, shake or oatmeal with protein powder
10% fat—avocado, nuts
10-15% fruit
Non-caloric beverage—tea or coffee without sugar or artificial sweetener

Lunch

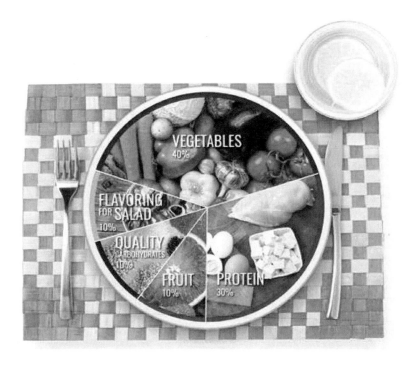

40% vegetables
30% protein
10% fruit
10% quality carbohydrates—grains, quinoa, beans or legumes
10% flavoring for salads or vegetables

Dinner

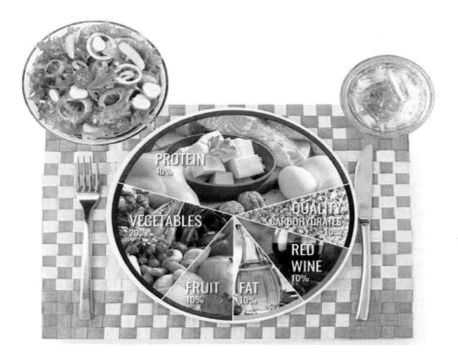

20% vegetables
40% protein
10% fruit
10% quality carbohydrates—grains, quinoa or legumes
10% fat—olive oil, avocado, etc.

Unlimited Vegetables
Enjoy up to 2 cups for lunch and dinner

Artichokes	Garlic
Arugula	Ginger
Asparagus	Jicama
Beans, yellow or green	Kale
Beets	Leeks
Bell Peppers	Lettuce
Bok Choy	Mushrooms
Broccoli	Okra
Brussels sprouts	Onions
Cabbage	Peas
Carrots	Peppers
Cauliflower	Radish
Celery	Snow peas
Chili peppers	Spinach
Collard greens	Sprouts
Cucumbers	Squash
Endive	Tomato
Eggplant	Turnips
Escarole	Watercress
Fennel	Zucchini

HEALTHY CARBOHYDRATES
Portion size 1/4 cup per day is preferred

GRAINS
Amaranth
Buckwheat groats (Kasha)
Brown Rice
Millet
Quinoa
Teff (grain from Ethiopia)
Wild Rice

VEGETABLES
Corn
Squash-summer & winter varieties
Sweet Potatoes
Water Chestnuts

BEANS
Black beans
Chickpeas (Garbanzo Beans)
Great Northern beans
Kidney beans
Lentils
Lima beans
Navy beans

Pinto beans
Soy Milk
Soy Yogurt
Soybeans and edamame
Split peas
Tofu
White beans (cannellini)

1 Week of Suggested Sample Menus

With **all** dinners, you may enjoy a large (2-3 cups) mixed salad with a splash of oil/balsamic vinegar or lemon juice

DAY 1

Breakfast	Eggs and egg whites with avocado
Snack	Carrot and celery sticks
Lunch	Roasted veggies with easy fried egg
Snack	Celery with nut dip of your choice: peanut, almond, cashew (1/4 C nonfat cream cheese mixed with a tsp. of nut butter).
Dinner	Cauliflower crusted pizza
	Large mixed green salad with oil/vinegar dressing

DAY 2

Breakfast	Protein pancakes
Snack	Healthy Kabob: 2 strawberries, 2 sq. of Swiss cheese and 4 cherry tomatoes or 2 cubes of jicama.
Lunch	Kale Salad, garlic and lemon dressing with pine nuts and raisins
Snack	2 tbsp. of hummus and veggies
Dinner	Zucchini Noodle Dish

DAY 3

Breakfast	Egg-white frittatas (pepper, onions, feta cheese & spinach)
Snack	½ avocado or 2 sticks of string cheese

Lunch	Mediterranean chicken (or tofu) lettuce wrap tacos
Snack	Medium apple sliced, with 10 raw almonds
Dinner	Shakshuka Dish

DAY 4

Breakfast	Cauliflower, cheese & eggs in cupcake cups
Snack	½ C Cottage cheese with 1/4 scoop of protein powder
Lunch	Mixed garden salad with 1/4 of avocado, 4 oz. sliced turkey, chicken or individual pack/can of water-packed tuna
Snack	Turkey/salmon jerky with veggies
Dinner	Light Eggplant Parmesan

DAY 5

Breakfast	Italian Baked Eggs and Vegetables
Snack	4 oz tomato, V8 juice
Lunch	½ C cottage cheese or yogurt with 1 C berries, 1/8 C unsalted nuts.
Snack	Babaghanoush with unlimited celery/cucumbers
Dinner	Salmon and Vegetable packets

DAY 6

Breakfast	Light Crustless Quiche
Snack	¼ C blueberries & 2 oz. of string cheese
Lunch	1 hard-boiled egg mixed with mustard
Snack	Dill pickles & sweet peppers
Dinner	Shrimp Catalan

DAY 7

Breakfast	Baked-Eggs-Avocado
Snack	Celery stuffed with nonfat cream cheese or cottage cheese (1/4 C)
Lunch	Tuna salad with celery & onions mixed with mustard over lettuce
Snack	2 slices of tomatoes with basil & shredded low fat mozzarella cheese
Dinner	Oven roasted chicken or fish 5 oz., veggies & salad

Power of 5 Recipes

Breakfast
High Protein Oatmeal

Servings 1
Prep 2 minutes
Cook 3 minutes
Total 5 minutes*
***Time will be slightly higher if using steel-cut oats as they take longer to cook. You may prepare them a day ahead of time.**

Ingredients:

- ¼-½C oatmeal, your choice of oats, rolled, quick or steel-cut; however, keep in mind to maintain a portion size that is no more than 150 calories.
- ½ C water
- 1 scoop fiber supplement (i.e. Benefiber)
- ½ scoop protein power of your choice and flavor (high protein/low carb preferred)

Instructions:
Cook oatmeal in microwave for one minute
    Add protein powder and fiber supplement
    Add 1-2 tbsp. milk (for added protein)

Nutritional information (1 Serving):
Calories: 245
Carbohydrates 27g
Fiber 6g
Fat 4g
Protein 28g
Sugar 3g

Protein Pancakes
Inspired by: Training4Fitness, adapted in the Power of 5 test kitchen

Servings 6
Prep 10 minutes
Cook 15 minutes
Total 25 minutes

Ingredients:

- ½ C high quality protein powder
- ½ C almond flour (or oats)
- ½ tsp. baking soda
- ¼ tsp. sea salt
- 10 drops liquid stevia (or half a banana)
- 4 eggs
- 1 C cottage cheese
- ½ C low fat milk
- 1 tbsp. coconut oil

Instructions:
Combine the protein powder, almond flour, baking soda and salt in a medium bowl. Mix until fully combined.

In a food processor combine the stevia, eggs, cottage cheese and milk. Add the dry ingredients and pulse to combine.

Heat a pancake griddle over medium heat. Grease with the coconut oil, cook the batter by ¼ C scoops until bubbles form, then flip and cook the other side until golden. Serve with grass-fed butter. Enjoy!

Nutritional Information (1 serving):
Calories 311
Carbohydrate 11g
Protein 37g
Fat 12g
Fiber 2g

Egg-White Frittata
Power of 5 test kitchen, adapted from popsugar.com
This is a delicious, filling breakfast, brunch or any meal.

Servings 2 large
Prep 10 minutes
Cook 10 minutes
Total 20 minutes

Ingredients:

- 2 tbsp. olive oil
- 1 red pepper, chopped
- 1 green pepper, chopped
- ¼ yellow onion, chopped
- 1 tsp. kosher salt
- 1 tsp. black pepper
- 8 egg whites (either separated or from a carton)
- ½ C feta cheese, crumbled
- 2 C fresh spinach

Instructions:
Preheat the oven to 375°F. (If you use whole eggs instead of egg whites, bake at 400°F)

In a heavy skillet, add olive oil and bring to medium-low heat.

Sauté onions and peppers until vegetables are tender, about 7 minutes.

Sprinkle the mixture with salt and pepper.

Pour egg whites into the skillet and cook for 3 minutes.

Sprinkle the top with feta and spinach.

Put skillet in oven and bake, uncovered, for 8 to 10 minutes.

Loosen the edges of the frittata with a rubber spatula, and then invert onto a plate.

Nutritional information: (1 serving)
Calories 333
Total Fat 22.6g
Saturated Fat 7.7g
Total Carbohydrates 11.9g
Dietary Fiber 3.5g
Sugars 7.1g
Protein 21.9g

Cook's Notes
This can also be made on top of the stove in a covered skillet once you have gathered all the ingredients together. Your preference!

Italian Baked Egg and Vegetables
Power of 5 test kitchen, inspired from www.popsugar.com

Servings 4
Prep 20 minutes
Cook 60 minutes
Total 80 minutes

Ingredients

- 1 pound plum tomatoes, cut into 1-in. chunks
- 1 red bell pepper, cut into 3/4-in. pieces
- 1 zucchini, quartered lengthwise, cut crosswise into 3/4-in. chunks
- 1 onion, halved lengthwise, sliced
- 2 large garlic cloves, minced
- 1/2 tsp. dried basil (or 1/2 tbs. fresh)
- 1/2 tsp. salt
- 1/4 tsp. black pepper
- 4 large eggs
- 1/4 C grated fat-free Parmesan cheese

Instructions

Heat oven to 400°F, and cover a shallow roasting pan with nonstick cooking spray. Put tomatoes, bell pepper, zucchini, onion, garlic, basil, salt, and pepper in pan and also spray with nonstick spray; toss to coat. Roast, stirring occasionally, until vegetables are browned and tender, about 30 minutes.

Spray four 8- or 10-ounce ramekins or custard cups with nonstick spray. Divide roasted vegetables evenly among cups. Make a well in the center of the vegetables, and carefully break one egg into each cup. Sprinkle with Parmesan cheese. Place cups on baking sheet, and bake until eggs are just set, 20 to 25 minutes.

Nutritional Information: (1 serving)

Calories 149
Total Fat 5.4g
Total Carbohydrates 13.7g
Dietary Fiber 3.1g
Sugars 8.2g
Protein 9.1g

Light Crustless Quiche
Power of 5 test kitchen, inspired by www.skinnymom.com

Servings 1 slice
Prep 10 minutes
Cook 50 minutes
Total 60 minutes

Ingredients:

- 1 C low-fat cottage cheese
- 2 C liquid egg whites
- ½ C broccoli, cooked and chopped
- ½ C extra lean ham, diced
- ½ C Reduced Fat Sharp Cheddar Shredded Cheese
- ¼ tsp. salt
- ¼ tsp. black pepper

Instructions:
Preheat oven to 375° F.
Mix all ingredients in a large mixing bowl.
Spray 9½-in. pie pan with nonstick cooking spray and pour ingredients in.
Bake for approximately 45 minutes or until center is set.

Nutrition Information: (1 serving = 1 slice)
Calories: 111
Carbohydrates: 3g
Protein: 15g
Fat: 3g
Fiber: 0g
Sugars: 1g

Baked-Eggs-Avocado
Power of 5 test kitchen, inspired by POPSUGAR.com Fitness

Servings: 4
Prep 8 minutes
Cook 20 minutes
Total 28 minutes

Ingredients:

- 2 ripe avocados
- 4 fresh eggs
- 1/8 teaspoon pepper
- 1 tbsp. chopped chives

Instructions
Preheat the oven to 425°F.

Slice the avocados in half and remove the pit. Scoop out about two tbsp. of flesh from the center of the avocado, just enough so the egg will fit snugly in the center.

Place the avocados in small, round individual baking dishes. Do your best to make sure they fit tightly.

Crack an egg into each avocado half. Try your best to crack the yolk in first, then let the egg whites spill in to fill the rest of the shell.

Place in the oven and bake for 15 to 20 minutes. Cooking time will depend on the size of your eggs and avocados. Just make sure the egg whites have enough time to set.

Remove from oven, then season with pepper, chives, and garnish of your choice.

Nutritional Information: (1 serving)
Serving Size 145g
Calories 268
Total Fat 24.0g
Total Carbohydrates 9.1g
Dietary Fiber 6.8g
Sugars 0.9g

Enjoy! This makes a lovely breakfast or brunch dish for company.

Cauliflower-Cheese-Egg Cupcakes
Power of 5 test kitchen, inspired by www.delish.com

Servings 12 cups
Prep 10 minutes
Cook 30 minutes
Total 40 minutes

Ingredients

- 2 heads of cauliflower, steamed
- 2 C shredded cheddar cheese
- 1 dozen + 2 large eggs
- 1 tsp. garlic powder
- 1 tsp. salt
- Fresh ground pepper to taste
- Chives, chopped (optional)
- Bacon bits (optional for bacon flavor or to keep it vegetarian.)

Instructions:
Preheat oven to 375° F. Lightly grease a 12-cup muffin tin and set aside.

Drop the steamed cauliflower into the bowl of a food processor and pulse until it resembles a fine grain.

Pour the ground cauliflower onto paper towels and twist to wring out excess liquid. Do this up to three times until the cauliflower comes out completely dry.

Transfer dry cauliflower to a large mixing bowl. Add cheddar cheese, garlic powder, salt and two eggs; stir to combine.

Distribute the mixture evenly throughout the muffin tins and use your fingers to press the mixture into the sides and bottom of each cup to form the nests.

Bake the nests for 15-17 minutes until brown.

Add a couple of bacon bits to the bottom of each cup and crack an egg on top, without breaking the yolk.

Bake for 7-8 minutes.

Sprinkle with chives and pepper to taste.

Nutrition Information: (1 Serving)
Serving Size 122 g
Calories 172
Total Fat 12.1g
Saturated Fat 5.8g
Total Carbohydrates 3.4g
Dietary Fiber 1.1g
Sugars 1.7g
Protein 13.0g

Lunch

Roasted Veggies with Easy Fried Egg
Power of 5 test kitchen, inspired by www.popsugar.com
Very easy

Makes 1 serving
Prep 15 minutes
Cook 20 minutes
Total 35 minutes

Ingredients

- Roasted veggies (you can add/delete veggies to taste)
- 1/2 large head cauliflower, cut into florets
- 2 small heads broccoli, cut into florets
- 1 1/2 tbsp. extra-virgin olive oil
- 1/4 tsp. garlic powder
- 1/4 tsp. salt
- 1/4 tsp. pepper
- 1/2 tsp. red pepper flakes
- Juice of 1/2 lemon
- Fried Egg
- Canola oil spray
- 1 egg
- Pinch of paprika, optional
- Dash of hot sauce, optional

Instructions
Preheat oven to 400° F.

In a large bowl, toss cauliflower and broccoli florets in extra-virgin olive oil. Then add the garlic powder, salt, pepper, and red pepper flakes, and mix well.

Spread out your veggies on a baking sheet and give all the florets a good squeeze of fresh lemon juice.

Roast in the oven for 15 to 20 minutes, occasionally shaking the pan.

Once your veggies have roasted for 10 to 12 minutes, heat a small nonstick skillet over medium-low heat, and give it a good spray of canola oil. Crack your egg in the skillet, and cook for about three minutes until the yolk is slightly set.

Remove your veggies from the oven and slide them into a shallow plate or bowl.

Flip your egg and cook for an additional 30 seconds to a minute. Keep the cook time shorter if you like a runny egg!

Carefully slide your cooked egg on top of your veggies, sprinkle with paprika, and eat up.

Nutritional Information: (1 serving)
Calories 349
Carbohydrates 19.4g
Fat 27.3g
Saturated fat 4.9g
Fiber 7.8g
Sugars 7.2g
Protein 12.8g

Kale Salad, Garlic and Lemon Dressing with Pine Nuts and Raisins
Power of 5 test kitchen, originally from Kale Cookbook
This is a delicious fresh Kale salad that can be adapted with a variety of ingredients to change it up.

Servings 12
Prep 18 minutes
Cook 0 minutes
Total 18 minutes

Ingredients:

- 4 bunches of leafy green kale, stems removed, chiffonade (chopping technique - leafy green vegetables are cut into long strips) or 1 bag of organic kale.

- 2 C grated Parmesan cheese
- 3 bunches of scallions (or to taste) finely chopped
- 2 C of currants (or 1 cup of raisins)
- 1-2 C toasted pine nuts. Carefully toast in a pan on low heat as they burn easily
- 1 C fresh-squeezed lemon juice
- 1 C extra virgin olive oil
- 2-3 cloves of chopped garlic
- Kosher salt. Pepper

Instructions:
Remove the center stems from the kale. Tear into bite-size pieces.
Mix olive oil, lemon juice and seasoning. Toss with combined ingredients.
Prepare 1 – 2hrs. before serving.
Keeps well for 1-2 days
I usually halve the recipe.

Options (not included in the list of ingredients):
Swap out pine nuts for slivered almonds or walnuts or 1/2 cup cooked quinoa!
Omit cheese.
Add cherry tomatoes or sliced tomatoes.
Add 5 oz. piece of protein: Tuna (150 calories), Salmon (240 calories) or Chicken (234 calories) on top, keeping in mind this will add to your total calories for this dish.

Nutritional Information: (1 serving)
Calories 248
Carbohydrates 5g
Fiber 1.5g
Sugar 8.2g
Protein 3.7g
Fat 25.3g

Additional notes
If you like Kale salad (it's a nightly staple in our house) give it a try! As you can see, you can adapt the recipe to your tastes. Remember: The dark leafy vegetables have wonderful benefits—rich in plenty of Vitamins K, A, and C.

Mediterranean Chicken (or Tofu) Lettuce Wrap Tacos
Power of 5 test kitchen, inspired by Martha Stewart.com
Substitute Tofu instead of chicken, use plant-based chicken, OR eliminate the meat altogether.

Servings 4
Prep 20 minutes
Cook 8 minutes
Total 28 minutes

Ingredients:

- 12 oz. boneless skinless chicken breasts, cut into 4-inch-long, 1-inch-thick strips OR replace with plain baked tofu cut in small squares.
- 2 tsp. Mediterranean spice
- 1 tbsp. dried basil
- 1 tbsp. dried oregano
- 1 tbsp. coarse salt
- 1 1/2 tsp. freshly ground black pepper
- 1/4 C balsamic vinaigrette
- 1/4 C balsamic vinegar
- 1/4 C red-wine vinegar
- 1 tbsp. soy sauce
- 1 1/2 tsp. chopped shallots
- 1 tbsp. plus 1 1/2 teaspoons Dijon mustard
- 1 tbsp. chopped garlic
- 1 tbsp. sugar
- 1 tsp. coarse salt
- 1 tsp. freshly ground black pepper
- 1 1/2 C olive oil
- 4 romaine lettuce leaves, shredded
- 1 tbsp. thinly sliced red onion
- 1/4 C red-wine vinaigrette
- 1/2 C red-wine vinegar
- 1/2 C balsamic vinaigrette

- 2 tsp. sugar
- 1 1/2 tsp. coarse salt
- 1 tsp. dried basil
- 1 tsp. dried oregano
- 1/4 tsp. freshly ground black pepper
- 1/4 C plus 2 tbsp. extra-virgin olive oil
- 1/4 C Tzatziki
- 1/2 finely chopped, peeled, and seeded cucumber
- Coarse salt
- 3/4 C Greek yogurt
- 1/4 C sour cream
- 5 fresh mint leaves, finely chopped
- Pinch sugar
- Pinch garlic powder
- 5 cilantro leaves, finely chopped
- 1 scallion, white and light green parts only, finely chopped
- Pinch freshly ground black pepper
- 12 butter lettuce leaves
- 4 Roma tomatoes, chopped
- 1 1/2 oz. crumbled feta cheese
- 12 Kalamata olives, pitted and chopped
- 1 tsp. chopped parsley
- 1/2 tsp. dried basil
- 1/2 tsp. dried oregano

Instructions:
Preheat a grill pan over high heat. Season chicken/tofu with 1 tsp. Mediterranean spice and place on grill. Cook, basting with balsamic vinaigrette and turning once, until cooked through, about 2 minutes per side. Season chicken/tofu with remaining tsp. Mediterranean spice and remove from grill; set aside.

Place shredded romaine lettuce and red onions in a medium bowl; drizzle with red-wine vinaigrette and toss to combine. Divide mixture evenly among butter lettuce leaves and drizzle each with 1 tsp. tzatziki.

Top each taco with 1 piece of chicken/tofu and garnish with chopped tomatoes, feta cheese, and olives. Season with parsley, basil, and oregano; serve.

Additional notes
Cook's Notes: This is a very versatile recipe that can easily be adapted based on your eating preferences.

Nutritional information: (1 serving)
Using Chicken
Calories 350
Carbohydrates 19g
Fat 0g
Protein 22g

Using Tofu
Calories 400
Carbohydrates 12g
Fat 3g
Protein 35g

Cottage Cheese (or Yogurt), Berries & Nuts
Prep 5 minutes
Cook 0 minutes
Total 5 minutes

Ingredients:

- ½ C low-fat cottage cheese or Greek plain yogurt
- 1 C berries,
- 1/8 C unsalted nuts

Instructions
Measure and combine all ingredients together in a bowl. Enjoy

Nutritional information: (1 serving)
Calories 262
Carbohydrates 24.5g
Fiber 4.6g
Protein 17g

A Simple Egg
Prep 5 minutes
Cook 0 minutes
Total 5 minutes

Ingredients:

- 1 hard-boiled egg
- Mustard

Instructions:
Place egg(s) in a 2-quart saucepan. Cover with cold water at least 1 inch above the eggs. Cover the saucepan and heat to boiling. Immediately remove from heat; let stand covered 15 minutes, then drain.

Immediately place eggs in cold water with ice cubes or run cold water over eggs until completely cooled.

Mustard may be used as a dipping sauce.

Nutritional Information:
Calories 83
Carbohydrates .6g
Protein 6g
Fiber 0g

Tuna Salad with Celery & Onions mixed with Mustard over Lettuce
Prep 10 minutes
Cook 0 minutes
Total 10 minutes

Ingredients:

- ¼ C tuna
- 2 stalks of celery, chopped
- 3 tbsp. chopped onions

- 1 tsp. mustard
- Lettuce leaves

Instructions:
Measure tuna in a bowl, chop celery and onions, add mustard and mix. Roll tuna mixture in a lettuce leaf and enjoy!

Nutritional information:
Calories 88
Carbohydrates 3g
Fat 1.5g
Protein 13.4g

Asparagus and Smoked Salmon Wraps
Prep 10 minutes
Cook 10 minutes
Total 20 minutes

Ingredients

- 1 bunch asparagus, ends trimmed (about 20 spears)
- 1 tbsp. olive oil
- Pinch kosher salt
- Pinch freshly ground black pepper
- 4 to 6 oz. thinly sliced smoked salmon

Instructions
Preheat oven to 400°F.

Lay the asparagus on a foil-lined baking sheet. Drizzle with olive oil and sprinkle with salt and pepper.

Roast until cooked and starting to brown around the edges, about 10 minutes. Remove from the oven and transfer to another baking sheet to cool.

Once the asparagus spears have cooled, wrap four or five spears together with one slice of smoked salmon. Repeat with the rest of asparagus spears and salmon slices.

Nutritional information:

Calories 265

Fat 8g

Carbohydrate 11.5g

Fiber 6g

Protein 38.3g

Dinner

Cauliflower Crusted Pizza

This delicious low-calorie and low-carbohydrate pizza is very satisfying and tasty!

Servings 2
Prep 30 minutes
Cook 15 minutes
Total 45 minutes

Ingredients:

- 1 medium-sized cauliflower head
- ¼ tsp. kosher salt
- ½ tsp. dried and crushed basil
- ½ tsp. dried and crushed oregano
- ½ tsp. garlic powder
- ¼ C shredded Parmesan cheese
- ¼ C mozzarella cheese
- 3-4 artichoke hearts (in water), chopped
- 1 egg

Toppings:
I have used all of these. All are delicious, but choose your preference!

Cherry tomatoes sliced in half
Thinly sliced onions
Thinly sliced mushrooms
Sliced avocados
Roasted red peppers

Alternatives:
Shrimp
Chicken
Tofu
Pepperoni or vegetarian sausage

Instructions:
Place your pizza stone/upside-down baking sheet in the oven and heat to 450F.

Trim the large green leaves and stems and roughly chop cauliflower into 2-inch pieces.

Rinse the cauliflower under running water.

Place the cauliflower in a food processor or blender. Pulse cauliflower until it looks like powdery snow. If your processor/blender is smaller, just grind the cauliflower in batches (or grate the cauliflower head the old-fashioned way – this will take longer).

Remove the ground cauliflower from the processor/blender and place in a microwave-safe bowl. Cover the bowl loosely with a paper towel or plastic wrap and microwave for 3 minutes.

Place the (hot!) ground cauliflower onto a dish towel and spread evenly so that it will cool down faster. After the cauliflower is cool enough to handle, gather it into a pile in the center of the dishtowel, gather the corners, and wring the water content out of the cauliflower over a sink. This is **VERY IMPORTANT:** spend a few minutes wringing out the water! Just one or two wrings will not get the job done. I spent more than 5 minutes on mine.

Empty the cauliflower from the dishtowel back into a bowl. Don't be alarmed if the amount of cauliflower without water fits in your hand—this is still enough to work with!

Mix the cauliflower with the mozzarella and Parmesan cheeses, the oregano, basil, kosher salt, and garlic powder and chopped artichokes.

When everything is mixed, add the egg and mix again until the egg is fully blended.

If you have a pizza paddle (called a peel), place parchment paper on the paddle. If not, a cutting board will still do the trick—just place your parchment paper on top of the board.

Dump the cauliflower mixture onto the parchment paper and form into a 12-in. diameter crust with a thickness of ¼ in. [**NOTE:** Be sure to grease well your parchment paper with olive oil spray, before placing the mixture, to ensure that the crust doesn't stick to the surface!]

Slide the parchment paper off your peel/board and onto the pizza stone/baking sheet in the oven and bake for 8-11 minutes, or until the crust is golden-brown and looks crispy at the edges.

Grab the parchment paper and slide it and the pizza crust back onto your peel/board, close the oven, and garnish with your chosen toppings.

Place the pizza and the parchment paper back into the oven and on the stone/sheet for another 5-7 minutes. My pizza finished baking in 5 minutes!

Let it cool down for a few minutes before slicing up and digging in.

Cook's Notes
I like my pizza crispy, so I increased the cooking time by a few minutes.

Nutritional Information: (1 serving = ½ of the pizza)
Calories 543
Carbohydrate 26.3g
Fat 29.2g
Fiber 7.1g
Sugar 9.8g
Protein 43.2g

Zucchini Noodles
Power of 5 test kitchen, inspired by Natalie Morales on *The Today Show*.

Servings 4
Prep 10 minutes
Cook 10 minutes
Total 20 minutes

Ingredients:
Zucchini noodles

- 4 yellow and green zucchini
- 1 tbsp. olive oil
- Salt and pepper, to taste
- ¼ C Parmesan cheese, plus more for topping

Vegetable sauté

- 1 tbsp. olive oil
- 4 Italian chicken (or veggie) sausages, chopped (optional)
- 1 C cherry tomatoes, sliced in half
- 1 6-oz. package cremini mushrooms, cleaned and chopped
- 2 cans cannellini beans
- ¼ onion, sliced
- Salt and pepper, to taste

Pesto

- 1 large clove garlic
- 3 C fresh basil
- ¼ C pine nuts
- ¼ C olive oil
- Salt and pepper, to taste

OPTIONAL *for Non-Meat Eaters*: replace the sausage with vegetable sausage or spiced up crumbles and get the same delicious flavors.

Instructions:
Cut the ends off the zucchini and put through a spiralizer (Veggetti and Paderno both make these handy spiral cutting tools) or use a manual vegetable peeler to get long spaghetti-like strands. Set aside.

Add garlic, basil, pine nuts and olive oil into a food processor.

Add salt and pepper to taste. Set aside.

Heat a skillet on medium heat and add 1 tbsp. of olive oil. Cook chicken sausage until browned, turning occasionally, about 8 minutes.

Add mushrooms, tomatoes and onions to sausage in the skillet.

Stir until combined. It will create almost a stew.

Once vegetables are cooked through, add beans and salt and pepper to taste.

Heat another large skillet and add a tbsp. of olive oil.

Once heated, add the zucchini noodles, stirring occasionally.

Sauté until zucchini is slightly softened, about 6 minutes.

Add pesto to zucchini and stir until noodles are evenly coated.
Add Parmesan cheese and a dash of salt, if desired. Lower the heat.
Put noodles in a large serving dish and top with vegetable mixture.
Give it a toss, and top with more Parmesan cheese, if desired

Nutritional Information: (1 serving)
Calories 519
Fat 33g
Carbohydrate 26.5g
Fiber 10.2g
Protein 28.15g

Cook's Note: Most pesto recipes call for you to add grated Parmesan at the
beginning, but I like to add it at the very end so you can really taste the cheese
and use less of it.

Shakshuka
Power of 5 test kitchen, inspired by toriavey.com

Servings 5-6
Prep 10 minutes
Cook 20 minutes
Total 30 minutes

Ingredients

- 1 tbsp. olive oil
- 1/2 medium brown or white onion, peeled and diced
- 1 clove garlic, minced
- 1 medium green or red bell pepper, chopped
- 4 C ripe diced tomatoes, or 2 cans (14 oz. each) diced tomatoes
- 2 tbsp. tomato paste
- 1 tsp. chili powder (mild)
- 1 tsp. cumin

- 1 tsp. paprika
- Pinch of cayenne pepper (or more, to taste—spicy!)
- Salt and pepper to taste
- 5-6 eggs
- 1/2 tbsp. fresh chopped parsley (optional, for garnish)

Instructions:
Heat a deep, large skillet or sauté pan on medium. Slowly warm olive oil in the pan. Add chopped onion; sauté for a few minutes until the onion begins to soften. Add garlic and continue to sauté till mixture is fragrant.

Add the bell pepper; sauté for 5-7 minutes over medium heat until softened.

Add tomatoes and tomato paste to pan; stir till blended. Add spices and sugar, stir well, and allow mixture to simmer over medium heat for 5-7 minutes till it starts to reduce. At this point, you can taste the mixture and spice it according to your preferences. Add salt and pepper to taste, more sugar for a sweeter sauce, or more cayenne pepper for a spicier Shakshuka (be careful with the cayenne...it is extremely spicy!).

Crack the eggs, one at a time, directly over the tomato mixture, making sure to space them evenly over the sauce. I usually place 4-5 eggs around the outer edge and 1 in the center. The eggs will cook "over easy" style on top of the tomato sauce.

Cover the pan. Allow mixture to simmer for 10-15 minutes, or until the eggs are cooked and the sauce has slightly reduced. Keep an eye on the skillet to make sure the sauce doesn't reduce too much, which can lead to burning.

Some people prefer their Shakshuka eggs more runny. If this is your preference, let the sauce reduce for a few minutes before cracking the eggs on top; then cover the pan and cook the eggs to taste.

Garnish with the chopped parsley, if desired. Shakshuka can be eaten for breakfast, lunch, or dinner. For breakfast, serve with warm, crusty bread or pita that can be dipped into the sauce (if you're gluten-intolerant or celebrating Passover, skip the bread). For dinner, serve with a green side salad for a light, easy meal.

Nutritional Information: (1Serving)
Calories 113
Carbohydrates 8.9g

Protein 6.4g
Fat 6.5g
Dietary Fiber 2.6g
Sugars 5.5g

Melissa's Famous Eggplant Parmesan

This has been a family & friend favorite for years. I have added low carb options.
Delicious either way! This recipe does take a bit of time to prepare, but is defi-
nitely worth it.

Servings: 4
Prep 35 minutes
Cook 1 hour, 20 minutes
Total 1 hour, 55 minutes

Ingredients

- 4 medium size eggplants (firm, fresh, no bruises) peeled, sliced into 1/2
  in. thick slices.
- 4-5 eggs (can use egg whites instead or mix with eggs to spread the
  dipping mixture)
- 1+ C Italian bread crumbs or Italian Pankos (you can forget the bread
  crumbs
- and place slices of eggplant on a cookie sheet seasoned with olive oil
  and layered with parchment paper).
- 1-2 C Shredded low-fat mozzarella cheese
- 1 1/2 C tomato sauce
- 2 tbsp. Parmesan cheese

Instructions

Once eggplant is prepared and sliced, salt both sides and let sit for 10 minutes,
then rinse off and pat dry with paper towels.
  Preheat oven to 425 °F
  In a medium size bowl, beat eggs and egg whites together.
  Place bread crumbs in another bowl.

Dip eggplant in eggs, then bread crumbs. Place on cookie sheet covered with greased parchment paper. Sprinkle olive oil lightly over top of eggplants. Do not drench.

Repeat until eggplant is all dipped/breaded and ready on the pan.

Bake 20 minutes or until side is brown (I like it crispy, myself.)

Flip and bake another 20 minutes on the other side. If you are using 2 pans of eggplant, you may have to shift them on your oven racks to get consistent cooking.

Once eggplant is cooked, let sit on paper towels to remove excess oil.

In a medium to large oven-safe casserole dish, layer eggplants with sauce then mozzarella cheese, then sauce, ending with cheese on top.

Sprinkle with the Parmesan cheese and bake for 20 minutes or until it bubbles.

Low Carb Version:
Use egg whites only

Omit the bread crumbs or Pankos

Season the paper- covered cookie sheet with garlic powder, salt, pepper, oregano, and basil, Place the eggplant on the sheet and season the top. Sprinkle with olive oil.

The eggplant will get soft and may not have a crispy exterior—not to worry.

Omit the cheese or use non-dairy cheese (non-dairy or vegan cheese does not melt as well as other cheeses).

Another option I have tried is no fat/low fat ricotta cheese mixed with an egg and garlic; spread on the eggplant, then layer with thinly sliced tomatoes (rather than tomato sauce). Layer until all eggplant, cheese substitute and tomatoes are used.

Bake for 20 minutes or until it bubbles.

Additional notes
Be sure to use a cookie sheet that has a lip on it.

Nutritional Information: (1 Serving)
Calories 350
Carbohydrates 8.9g

Protein 6.4g
Fat 6.5g
Fiber 2.6g
Sugars 5.5g

Salmon and Vegetables Packet
Power of 5 test kitchen, inspired by www.justasdelish.com

Makes 2 servings
Prep 5 minutes
Cook 20 minutes
Total 25 minutes

Ingredients

- 2 pieces (4-6 oz) skinless salmon fillets
- 1 fennel bulb, sliced paper thin (a mandolin slicer works best)
- 4 French beans
- 4 cherry tomatoes, halved
- 8 very thin lemon slices
- 1 tbsp. lemon juice
- Sea salt
- Freshly ground black pepper
- 2 long, rectangular baking papers

Instructions:
Preheat oven to 225°C (450°F).

Fold a baking paper in half to create a crease, and then open it up again. Place several slices of fennel bulb above the crease of the paper and sprinkle with salt. Place one fillet of salmon on top of the fennel bulb slices, beans and tomatoes on the side. Squeeze lemon juice over the ingredients and sprinkle generously with lemon zest, salt and pepper. Lay 3-4 thin slices of lemon over salmon.

Fold the parchment over the salmon and securely close. Seal the parchment paper well by repeatedly folding little sections over each other around the edges, taking care to make sure it is well sealed.

Place on a baking tray and bake for 10 minutes.

Serve packets on individual plates immediately. Open up the folded packet or cut open the middle to enjoy the meal.

Nutritional Information: (1 serving)
Calories 285.5
Carbohydrates 19g
Fiber 7.6g
Sugar 0g
Protein 42g

Shrimp Catalan
Power of 5 test kitchen, inspired by Pamela Izquierdo
One of the most popular and classic tapas. Shrimp is sautéed in olive oil and lots of garlic (2 "must-have" ingredients in Spanish cooking)

Makes 2 servings
Prep 10 minutes
Cook 8 minutes
Total 18 minutes

Ingredients

- 10-12 large shrimp, deveined. Can be cooked in shell or peeled.
- 3 cloves garlic, thinly sliced
- 1 tsp. lemon juice
- 2 tbsp. extra virgin olive oil
- Sea salt to taste
- 1 tsp. chopped fresh parsley
- 2 tbsp. extra virgin olive oil
- 1 small red apple, peeled and cut into ¼-in. cubes (can substitute peach or pear for apple)
- 3 tbsp. pine nuts
- large bag of fresh baby spinach (or kale/spinach mix)
- Sea salt to taste

Instructions
Sauté shrimp with garlic, oil, and lemon juice. Add sea salt/pepper.
Add additional oil, spinach, apples and pine nuts. Sauté until done.

Nutritional Information:
Calories 295
Carbohydrates 12g
Fiber 4g
Protein 11g

Additional notes
May be served with ¼ C cooked quinoa, black or brown rice, or black beans.

Oven Roasted Chicken with Veggies

Serves 2
Prep 15 minutes
Cook 30 minutes
Total 45 minutes

Ingredients:

- 2 whole chicken legs, About one pound chicken legs or breasts.
- 3/4 pound small boiling potatoes
- 1 red bell pepper
- 1 medium onion
- 1 tbsp. olive oil
- 1/2 tsp. dried thyme, crumbled
- 1 bunch arugula (about 2 packed cups)
- 1/4 C dry white wine

Instructions:
Preheat oven to 450°F. Cut whole chicken legs into thighs and drumsticks and pat dry. Halve potatoes. Cut bell pepper into 1/2-inch-wide strips and onion into 1/2-inch-thick wedges.

In a large, flameproof roasting pan toss chicken, potatoes, bell pepper, and onion with oil, thyme, and salt and pepper to taste until coated; arrange in one layer, chicken skin side up.

Roast chicken and vegetables 30 minutes, or until chicken is cooked through and golden.

While chicken and vegetables are roasting, discard any coarse stems from arugula and put arugula in a large bowl.

With tongs transfer chicken and vegetables to bowl with arugula. Add wine to pan and deglaze over moderately high heat, stirring and scraping up brown bits for about a minute.

Pour sauce over chicken and vegetables. Toss and divide between two plates.

Nutritional Information: (1 serving)
Calories 369
Fat 21.5g
Carbohydrates 0g
Fiber 3g
Protein 0g

Cook's Note: Fish of your choice or plant-based protein may be substituted for chicken.

Snacks

100 Calories or less
1 oz. of Mozzarella Part-skim String Cheese
Calories 70
Fat 4.5g
Carbohydrates 1g
Fiber 0g
Protein 6g

Celery stuffed with low fat cottage cheese
½ C of cottage cheese (low fat)
2 stalks of Celery

Calories 90
Fiber 0g
Carbohydrates 4g
Fiber 0g
Protein 14g

Cucumber "boats" filled with tuna salad
Medium size cucumber, peeled, seeds scooped out of center
¼ C tuna in water mixed with mustard

Calories 100
Carbohydrates 0g
Fiber 0g
Fat 1.5g
Protein 13g

Haas Avocado (small)
1/3 Avocado

Calories 100
Fat 9.8g

Carbohydrates 1.2g
Fiber 4.5
Protein 1.3g

1 oz. Beef or Turkey Jerky (cured without sugar)
This makes an easy, low cal, on-the-go snack. There are many varieties. Just be sure they are not cured with sugar. You many even find salmon jerky as well.

Calories 80
Fat 1g
Carbohydrates 1g
Fiber 4g
Protein 12g

A Deviled Egg
Place egg in saucepan and cover with cold water; bring to a boil, cover and let sit for 15 minutes. Then run under cold water until cooled. Slice egg length-wise. Remove yolk and mix with 1 tsp. of mustard and 1 tsp. of light mayo; place back into egg- white casing and enjoy!

Calories 98
Fat 6.8g
Carbohydrates 1.1g
Fiber 1g
Protein 6.2g

Sliced Ham/Turkey rolled around a few raw or cooked green beans
Ham, turkey or chicken slices (2 oz.) and up to ½ C of green beans

Calories 100
Fat 2.2g
Carbohydrates 5.5g
Fiber 1.4g
Protein 10.5g

Two slices of tomato topped with chopped fresh basil and grated mozza-rella and run under the broiler for a minute
Calories 90
Fat 4g
Carbohydrates 1.7g
Fiber .8g
Protein 6.7g

½ C of unsweetened Greek yogurt mixed with 2 tbsp. no-added-sugar grated coconut
Calories 99
Fat 2.7g
Carbohydrate 4.6g
Fiber 3.3g
Protein 10.1g

Celery sticks dipped in peanut or another nut or seed butter
Calories 100
Fat 9.5g
Carbohydrates 3g
Flber .8g
Protein 2.5g

Cucumber "boats" filled with ricotta and sprinkled with seasoned salt
Peel & scoop out seeds of cucumber. Add ricotta and sprinkle with seasoning of your choice.

Calories 85
Fat 2.8g
Carbohydrates 10.3g
Fiber 1.4g
Protein 5.3g

Chunks of melon wrapped in slices of ham or smoked salmon
Cut 1/8 melon into chunks. Wrap each with 1 oz. of ham or smoked salmon

Calories 100
Fat 4.4g
Carbohydrates 10.1g
Fiber 1.2g
Protein 7.1g

"Kebab" of strawberries, pieces of light Swiss cheese, and cubes of jicama or celery.
½ C strawberries sliced in half, 2 pieces of Laughing Cow Cheese with pieces of jicama

Fat 8.2g
Carbohydrate 4.6g
Fiber 2g
Protein .6g

Cottage cheese topped with no-sugar-added salsa
½ C of fat-free cottage cheese, 4 tbsp. of salsa

Calories 96
Fat 0g
Carbohydrate 12g
Fiber 0g
Protein 12g

Mix 4 oz. tomato juice and 1 tbsp. sour cream in a bowl. Top with chunks of avocado, if desired.
Calories 81
Carbohydrate 30.4g
Fiber 2.3g
Protein 1.9g

¼ C Blueberries and a piece of string cheese.
Calories 100

Fat 6.1g
Carbohydrate 5.3g
Fiber .9g
Protein 6.3g

Fresh fruit salad with plain Greek yogurt, sprinkle of nuts
¼ C fruit salad, 3 tbsp. plain Greek yogurt, 2 tsp. unsalted nuts (preferably raw)

Calories 99
Fat 3.1g
Carbohydrates 6.7g
Fiber 1g
Protein 1.8g

Red or purple grapes with sliced turkey
½ C of grapes; 2 oz. of sliced turkey

Calories 100
Fat .5g
Carbohydrate15.5g
Fiber .7g
Protein 9g

Apple with raw almonds
½ small apple; 8 raw almonds

Calories 94
Fat 4.9g
Carbohydrate 9.4g
Fiber 3g
Protein 2.2g

Hummus with Raw Vegetables
2 tbsp. hummus, 4 baby carrots, 3 sweet peppers, 4 pieces celery

Calories 100
Fat 2.8g
Carbohydrates 10.7g
Fiber 4.6g
Protein 4.1g

Babaghanoush (eggplant dip) with vegetables—unlimited celery or cucumbers
1 tbsp. of dip with unlimited veggies

Calories 85
Fat 5.2g
Carbohydrates1.5g
Fiber 0g
Protein 0g

Skinny Popcorn, Homemade
2 ½ C, popped

Calories 100
Fat 6.7g
Carbohydrate 8g
Fiber 2g
Protein 1.3g

Carrot & celery sticks
1 C carrots; 4 celery stalks

Calories 79
Fat .5g
Carbohydrate 12.3g
Fiber 6g
Protein 2.4g

Part 1-Introduction

1. Davis, K., Stremikis, K. Schoen, C. and Squires, D. (2014, June) Mirror, Mirror on the Wall, 2014 Update: How the U.S. Health Care System Compares Internationally, The Commonwealth Fund.

2. Thompson, D. (2012, March). 10 Ways to Visualize How Americans Spend Money on Health Care. The Atlantic.

3. Hare, E. (2016, July 31). Life Expectancy. Retrieved February 12, 2017, from https://erikhare.com/2016/08/01/progress-and-history/

4. Thompson, D. (2012, March).

Chapter 1-The Power of 5

5. Health Risks. (2016, April 13). https://www.hsph.harvard.edu/obesit-prevention-source/obesity-consequences/health-effects/.

6. Lee, C. (2011, April 20). Right lifestyle choices will keep aging brain healthy. Retrieved February 12, 2016, from http://newsroom.ucla.edu/stories/right-lifestyle-choices-will-keep-201857.

7. Anand, P., Kunnumakara, A. B., Sundaram, C., Harikumar, K. B., Tharakan, S. T., Lai, O. S., . . . Aggarwal, B. B. (2008). Cancer is a Preventable Disease that Requires Major Lifestyle Changes. Pharmaceutical Research, 25(9), 2097-2116. doi:10.1007/s11095-008-9661-9.

8. Anand, P., et al., 2008, 2097-2116.

9. Lichtenstein, P., Holm, N.V., Verkasalo, P.K., Iliadou, A., Kaprio, J., Koskenvuo, M., Pukkala, E., Skytthe, A., Hemminki, K., (2000, July 13) Environmental and heritable factors in the causation of cancer--analyses of cohorts of twins

from Sweden, Denmark, and Finland. New England Journal of Medicine; 343(2):78-85.

10. Loeb, K.R., Loeb, L.A. (2000, March) Significance of multiple mutations in cancer. Carcinogenesis (3):379-85.

11. Hahn, W.C., Weinberg, R.A. (2002, May) Modeling the molecular circuitry of cancer. Nature Reviews Cancer; 2(5):331-41.

12. Mucci, L.A., Wedren, S., Tamimi, R.M., Trichopoulos, D., Adami, H.O. (2001, June) The role of gene-environment interaction in the aetiology of human cancer: examples from cancers of the large bowel, lung and breast, Journal of Internal Medicine; 249(6):477-93.

13. Czene, K., Hemminki, K. (2002, May) Kidney cancer in the Swedish Family Cancer Database: familial risks and second primary malignancies., Kidney International; 61(5):1806-1.

14. 2014 Surgeon General's Report: The Health Consequences of Smoking—50 Years of Progress. (2015, July 22). Retrieved February 12, 2016, from https://www.cdc.gov/tobacco/data_statistics/sgr/50th-anniversary/index.htm.

15. Cancer Facts & Figures 2010. (2010). Retrieved January 12, 2016, from https://www.cancer.org/research/cancer-facts-statistics/all-cancer-facts-figures/cancer-facts-figures-2010.html.

16. Secondhand Smoke and Cancer. (2011, January). Retrieved January 1, 2016, from https://www.cancer.gov/about-cancer/causes-prevention/risk/tobacco/second-hand-smoke-fact-sheet.

17. Anand, P., et al., 2008, 2097-2116.

18. Doll, R., Peto, R., (198, June) The causes of cancer: quantitative estimates o avoidable risks of cancer in the United States today. Journal of the National Cancer Institute; 66(6):1191-308

19. Willett, W.C. (2000) Diet and cancer. Oncologist; 5(5):393-404.

20. Anand, P., et al., 2008, 2097-2116.

21. Calle, E.E., Rodriguez, C., Walker-Thurmond, K., Thun, M.J. (2003, April 24) Overweight, obesity, and mortality from cancer in a prospectively studied cohort of U.S. adults. New England Journal of Medicine. 348(17): 1625-38.

22. Drewnowski, A., Popkin, B.M. (1997, Feb) The nutrition transition: new trends in the global diet. Nutrition Reviews. 55(2):31-43.

23. Hursting, S.D., Lashinger, L.M., Colbert, L.H., Rogers, C.J., Wheatley, K.W., Nunez, N.P., Mahabir, S., Barrett, J.C., Forman, M.R., Perkins, S.N. (2007, Aug) Energy balance and carcinogenesis: underlying pathways and targets for intervention. Current Cancer Drug Targets; 7(5):484-9.

24. Pisani, P., Parkin, D.M., Muñoz, N., Ferlay, J. (1997, June) Cancer and infection: estimates of the attributable fraction in 1990. Cancer Epidemiol Biomarkers Prev.; 6(6):387-400.

25. Parkin, D.M. The global health burden of infection-associated cancers in the year 2002. International Journal of Cancer: 2006 Jun 15; 118(12):3030-44.

26. De Maria, N., Colantoni, A., Fagiuoli, S., Liu, G.J., Rogers, B.K., Farinati, F., Van Thiel, D.H., Floyd, R.A.(1996) Association between reactive oxygen species and disease activity in chronic hepatitis C. Free Radical Biology and Medicine; 21(3):291-5.

27. Koike, K., Tsutsumi, T., Fujie, H., Shintani, Y., Kyoji, M..(2002) Molecular mechanism of viral hepatocarcinogenesis. Oncology. 62 Suppl 1():29-37.

28. The multitude and diversity of environmental carcinogens. Belpomme D, Irigaray P, Hardell L, Clapp R, Montagnier L, Epstein S, Sasco AJ. Environ Res. 2007 Nov; 105(3):414-29.(29) Guan, Y.S., He, Q., Wang, M.Q., Li, P. (2008 March) Nuclear factor kappa B and hepatitis viruses. Expert Opinion on Therapeutic Targets; 12(3):265

30. Belpomme, D. et al (2007). 414-29.

31. Divisi, D., Di Tommaso, S., Salvemini, S., Garramone, M., Crisci, R. (2006, Aug) Diet and Cancer., Acta Biomed. 77(2):118-23.

32. Steinmetz, K.A., Potter, J.D. (1996, Oct) Vegetables, fruit, and cancer prevention: a review. Journal of the American Dietetic Association 96(10):1027-39.

33. Green Anand, P., et al., 2008, 2097-2116wald, P. (2005) Lifestyle and medical approaches to cancer prevention. Recent Results in Cancer 166:1–15.

34. Vainio, H., Weiderpass, E. (2006) Fruit and vegetables in cancer prevention., Nutrition and Cancer. 54(1):111-42.

35. Divisi, D. et al, 2006, 118-23

36. Vainio, H. et al, 2006, 111-42

37. Wattenberg, L.W. (1966, July) Chemoprophylaxis of carcinogenesis: a review, Cancer Research. 26(7):1520-6.

38. Divisi, D, et al, 2006, 11-42.

39. Vainio, H. et al 2006, 11-42.

40. Anand, P., et al., 2008, 2097-2116.

41. Anand, P., et al., 2008, 2097-2116.

42. Booth, F.W., Chakravarthy, M.V., Gordon, S.E., Spangenburg, E.E. (2002, July), Waging war on physical inactivity: using modern molecular ammunition against an ancient enemy. Journal of Applied Physiology (1985). 93(1):3-30.

Chapter 2-Sweets

43. WHO (2016, June), Obesity and overweight fact sheet, updated

44. Binkley, J. K., , Eales, J. and Jekanowski, M. (2000), The relation between dietary change and rising US obesity, International Journal of Obesity 24, 1032-1039.

45. National Center for Health Statistics. Health, United States (2009): With Special Feature on Medical Technology. Hyattsville, MD. 2010.

46. National Center for Health Statistics. Health, United States (2009).

47. Colditz, G.A., Willett, W.C., Rotnitzky, A., Manson, J.E. (1995) Weight gain as a risk factor for clinical diabetes mellitus in women. Annals of Internal Medicine. 122:481–6.

48. Koh-Banerjee, P., Wang Y., Hu, F.B., Spiegelman, D., Willett, W.C., Rimm, E.B.(2004). Changes in body weight and body fat distribution as risk factors for clinical diabetes in US men. American Journal of Epidemiology. 159:1150–9.

49. Health Risks. (2016, April 13). https://www.hsph.harvard.edu/obesit-prevention-source/obesity-consequences/health-effects/.

50. Bogers, R.P., Bemelmans, W.J., Hoogenveen RT, et al. (2007) Association of overweight with increased risk of coronary heart disease partly independent of blood pressure and cholesterol levels: a meta-analysis of 21 cohort studies including more than 300,000 persons. Archives of Internal Medicine. 167:17208.

51. McGee, D.L. , (2005) mass index and mortality: a meta-analysis based on person-level data from twenty-six observational studies. Annals of Epidemiology 5:8797.

52. Strazzullo, P., Delia, L., Cairella, G., Garbagnati, F., Cappuccio, F.P., Scalfi, L. (2010) Excess body weight and incidence of stroke: meta-analysis of prospective studies with 2 million participants. Stroke. 41:e41826.

53. American Institute for Cancer Research, World Cancer Research Fund. (2007) Food, nutrition, physical activity and the prevention of cancer. Washington, D.C.: American Institute for Cancer Research.

54. Guh DP, Zhang W, Bansback N, Amarsi Z, Birmingham CL, Anis AH. (2009) The incidence of co-morbidities related to obesity and overweight: a systematic review and meta-analysis. BMC Public Health; 9:88.

55. Howard, Barbara V. , Van Horn, Linda, Hsia, Judith, (2006) Low-fat dietary pattern and risk of cardiovascular disease: the Women's Health Initiative Randomized Controlled Dietary Modification Trial -JAMA. 295(6): 655-666

56. de Wit, L., Luppino, F., van Straten, A., Penninx. B, Zitman, F., Cuijpers, P. (2010) Depression and obesity: a meta-analysis of community-based studies. Psychiatry Research. 178:2305.

57. Luppino, F.S., de Wit, L.M., Bouvy, P.F., et al. (2010) Overweight, obesity, and depression: a systematic review and meta-analysis of longitudinal studies. Archives of General Psychiatry. 67:2209.

58. McClean, K.M., Kee, F., Young, I.S., Elborn, J.S., (2008) Obesity and the lung: 1. Epidemiology.Thorax. 63:64954.

59. Alzheimers Association. Alzheimer's Facts and Figures. Alzheimers & Dementia. (2010); 6. Accessed January 25, 2012.

60. Beydoun. M.A., Beydoun, H.A., Wang, Y.(2008) Obesity and central obesity as risk factors for incident dementia and its subtypes: a systematic review and meta-analysis. Obesity Reviews 9:204-18

61. National Heart, Lung, and Blood Institute (2002). Clinical Guidelines on the Identification, Evaluation, and Treatment of Overweight and Obesity in Adults. Accessed January 25, 2012.

62. Esposito, K., Ciotola, M., Giugliano, F., Bisogni, C., Schisano, B., Autorino, R., . . . Giugliano, D. (2007, February 08). Association of body weight with

sexual function in women. Retrieved March 01, 2016, from http://www.nature.com/ijir/journal/ v19/ n4/ full/3901548a.html.

Chapter 3-Sweat

63. Moore, S.C., Patel, A.V., Matthews, C.E., Berrington de Gonzalez, A., Park, Y., Katki, H.A., et al. (2012) Leisure Time Physical Activity of Moderate to Vigorous Intensity and Mortality: A Large Pooled Cohort Analysis. PLoS Med 9(11): e1001335. doi:10.1371/journal.pmed.1001335

64. Haskell, W.L., Lee, I.M., Pate, R.R., Powell, K.E., Blair, S.N., Franklin, B.A., Macera, C.A., Heath, G.W., Thompson, P.D., Bauman, A. (2007, Aug) Physical activity and public health: updated recommendation for adults from the American College of Sports Medicine and the American Heart Association. Medicine & Science in Sports & Exercise 39(8):1423-34.

65. Arem, H., Moorse, S.C., Patel, A. Hartge, P., Berrington de Gonzalez, A., Visvanathan, K., Campbell, P.T., Freedman, M., Weiderpass, E., Adami, HQ, Linet, M.S., Matthews, C.E., (2015, June) Leisure time physical activity and mortality: a detailed pooled analysis of the dose-response relationship. JAMA Intern Med: Jun;175(6):959-67.

66. Srikanthan, Preethi, Karlamangla, Arun S., Preethi Srikanthan, Arun S. Karlamangla, Srikanthan P, Karlamangla (2014, February) A Muscle Mass Index As a Predictor of Longevity in Older Adults, American Journal of Medicine, Vol 127, Issue 6, Pgs. 547–553.

67. Ratey, John J., Hagerman, Eric (2013, Jan 1) SPARK The Revolutionary New Science of Exercise and the Brain. Little, Brown and Company; Reprint edition.

68. Ratey, John J. et al, 2013, Jan 1.

69. Ratey, John J. et al, 2013, Jan 1.

70. Hayley, Shawn, Littljohn, Shawn, Litteljohn, Darcy.(2013) Neuroplasticity and the next wave of antidepressant strategies. Frontiers in Cellular Neuroscience 7: 218.

71. Cooney, G.M., Dwan K, Greig C.A., Lawlor, D.A., Rimer, J., Waugh, F.R., McMurdo, M., Mead, G.E.(2013). Exercise for depression. Cochrane Database of Systematic Reviews, Issue 9.

72. Opezzo, Marily, Schwartz, Daniel L. (2014) Give Your Ideas Some Legs: The Positive Effect of Walking on Creative Thinking Journal of Experimental Psychology: Learning, Memory, and Cognition, Vol. 40, No. 4, 1142–1152

73. Diabetes and Physical Activity, National Institute of Diabetes and Digestive and Kidney Diseases.

74. President's Council on Fitness, Sports & Nutrition. (n.d.). Retrieved Oct. 05, 2016, from https://www.fitness.gov/be-active/physical-activity-guidelines-for-americans/.

75. How Exercise Can Help You. (2016, August 23). Retrieved Nov. 05, 2016, from https://go4life.nia.nih.gov/how-exercise-can-help-you.

76. Hoffmann, K., Frederiksen, K.S., Sobol, N.A., Beyer, N., Vogel, A., Simonsen, A.H., Johannsen, P., Lolk, A., Terkelsen, O., Cotman, C.W., Hasselbalch, S.G., Wald, (2013) Preserving cognition, quality of life, physical health and functional ability in Alzheimer's disease: the effect of physical exercise (ADEX trial): rationale and design. Neuroepidemiology. 41(3-4):198-207.

77. Liu-Ambrose, Teresa, Davis, Jennifer, Best, John R., Eng, Janice J., Lee, Philip E., Jacova, Claudia, Munkacsy, Michelle, Boyd, Lara, Hsiung, Robin, Ging-Yuek (2015, July) Vascular cognitive impairment and aerobic exercise: A 6-month randomized controlled trial Alzheimer's and Dementia The Journal of the Alzheimer's Association Vol 11, Issue 7, Supplement, Pgs. P323–P324.

78. Physical Activity and Cancer. (n.d.). Retrieved March 05, 2016, from https://www.cancer.gov/about-cancer/causes-prevention/risk/obesity/physical-activity-fact-sheet.

79. Arem, H., et al (2015 Jun) 175 (6):959-67.

80. Gerontoukou, Evangelia-Ioanna, Michaelidoy, Sofia, Rekleiti, Maria, Saridi, Maria and Souliotis, Kyriakos (2015, Sept. 30) Investigation of Anxiety and Depression in Patients with Chronic Diseases Health Psychology Research 3(2): 2123.

81. Chimkode, S.M., Kumaran, S.D., Kanhere, V.V., Shivanna, R. (2015, Apr) Effect of yoga on blood glucose levels in patients with type 2 diabetes mellitus. Journal of Clinical and Diagnostic Research 9(4).

82. The findings were presented at the Anxiety and Depression Association of America (ADAA) Conference 2015.

83. Kiecolt-Glaser, JK., Bennett, JM, Andridge, R, Peng J., Shapiro, CL. (2014), Yoga's impact on inflammation, mood, and fatigue in breast cancer survivors: a randomized controlled trial. Journal of Clinical Oncology 32 (10), 1040-1049.

84. Gonzalez-Wallace, M. (2012). Super body, super brain: the workout that does it all. New York: Harper One.

85. Bickel, C.S., Cross, J.M., Bamman, M.M. (2011, July) Exercise dosing to retain resistance training adaptations in young and older adults. Medicine & Science in Sports & Exercise 43(7):1177-87.

Chapter 4-Stress

86. Benson, H., Klipper, M. Z. (1975). The relaxation response. New York, NY: Harper Collins.

87. Administration on Aging, U.S. Department of Health and Human Services 2010 Population. Retrieved from www.aoa.gov/agingstatsdotnet/ Main_Site/Data/2010.

88. Jaskelioff M, et al. (2001) Telomerase reactivation reverses tissue degeneration in aged telomerase-deficient mice. Nature. 469:102-107.

89. Eisenberg, D.T.A. (2011) An evolutionary review of human telomere biology: the thrifty telomere hypothesis and notes on potential adaptive paternal effects. American Journal of Human Biology. 23:149–167.

90. Aubert, G., Lansdorp, P.M. (2008) Telomeres and aging. Physiological Reviews. 2008; 88:557–579.

91. Telomeres and Aging - Telomere Shortening. (n.d.). Retrieved Nov. 05, 2016, from https://www.tasciences.com/telomeres-and-cellular-aging/.

92. Effros, Rita B., (2011Feb-Mar) Telomere/telomerase dynamics within the human immune system: effect of chronic infection and stress. Experimental 46(2-3): 135–140.

93. Biology of Aging (2011, Nov) (updated 2015, Jan 22), National Institute on Aging, https://www.nia.nih.gov/health/publication/biology-aging/aging-under-microscope.

94. Biology of Aging, et al, (2011, Nov) (updated 2015, Jan. 22).

95. Biology of Aging, et al (2011, Nov) (updated 2015, Jan. 22).

96. Traustadottir, T. et al. (2005, May) The HPA axis response to stress in women: effects of aging and fitness. Psychoneuroendocrinology. 30(4): 392-402.

97. University of California at San Francisco (2004). Aging, the stress response, cortisol, and cognitive function.

98. Woolston, C. (March 2015) Aging and Stress. https://comsumer.healthday.com//encyclopedia//aging-1//age-health-news-7//aging-and-stress-645997.html.

99. Wilson, R.S. et al. (2003, Dec 9) Proneness to psychological distress is associated with Alzheimer's disease. Neurology. 61(11): 1479-1485.

100. Cohen, Sheldon, Janicki-Deverts, Denise, Gregory E. (2007, Oct 10) Psychological Stress and Disease, JAMA, Vol 298, No. 14 pp 1685-1687.

101. Gerontoukou, Evangelia-Ioanna, Michaelidoy, Sofia, Rekleiti, Maria, Saridi, Maria and Souliotis, Kyriakos (2015, Sep 30) Investigation of Anxiety and Depression in Patients with Chronic Diseases Health Psychol Res. 3(2): 2123.

102. Wilson, R.S., Schneider, J.A. et al. (2007) Chronic distress and incidence of mild cognitive impairment. Neurology 68:2085-2092.

103. Brodaty, Henry, Donkin, Marika (2009, Jun) Family caregivers of people with dementia Dialogues in Clinical Neuroscience 11(2): 217–228.

104. Schulz, R., Beach, S.R. (1999) Caregiving as a risk factor for mortality: The caregiver health effects study. JAMA 282:2215–2219.

105. Stress in America™ (2012, Jan 11): Our Health at Risk Stress, American Psychological Association.

106. Benson, H. et al, 1975.

107. Benson, H. et al, 1975.

108. Progressive Muscle Relaxation for Stress and Insomnia (2016 January 16) WebMD Medical Reference Reviewed by William Blahd, MD.

109. Arthritis Foundation, A Simple Exercise to Help You Relax in Ten Steps http://www.arthritis.org/living-with-arthritis/exercise/workouts/simple-routines/.

Chapter 5-Sleep

110. Office of Communications and Public Liaison National Institute of Neurological Disorders and Stroke, National Institutes of Health, Brain Basics: Understanding Sleep.

111. National Institute of Health (NIH), retrieved (2016, June) https://www.ninds.nih.gov/Disorders/Patient-Caregiver-Education/Understanding-Sleep.

112. Colten, H.R., Altevogt, B.M.-editors (2006) Sleep Disorders and Sleep Deprivation: An Unmet Public Health Problem. Institute of Medicine (US) Committee on Sleep Medicine and Research; Washington (DC): National Academies Press (US).

113. National Center for Chronic Disease and Prevention and Health Promotion, Division of Adult and Community Health.

114. National Institute of Health (NIH), retrieved (2016, June) from https://www.ninds.nih.gov/Disorders/Patient-Caregiver- Education/Understanding-Sleep.

115. Harvard Health Publications, Harvard Medical School: Sleep Medication Table, retrieved (2016, June) from http://www.health.harvard.edu/newsletter_article/medications-that-can-affect-sleep.

116. National Sleep Foundation: www.ninds.nih.gov: Adapted from "When You Can't Sleep: The ABCs of ZZZs," published by the National Sleep Foundation https://sleepfoundation.org.

Chapter 6-Sex

117. Pfeifer, Eric. (1972) Determinants of Sexual Behavior: Middle and Old Age. Journal of the American Geriatrics Society: Vol. 20. pp. 151-158.

118. U. S. Census Bureau. (2005, Dec) 65+ in the United States.

119. AARP. (1999) Modern Maturity Sexuality Survey, Washington, DC: National Family Opinion (NFO) Research.

120. Leary, W. (1998, Sept) Older People Enjoy Sex, Survey Says. New York Times, Retrieved 2016, http://www.nytimes.com/1998/09/29/science/older-people-enjoy-sex-survey-says.html.

121. Westheimer, R.K., Lehu, P.A. (2005) Dr. Ruth's sex after 50: revving up the romance, passion and excitement! Sanger, CA: Quill Driver Books/Word Dancer Press.

RESOURCES

BMI; using the National Heart, Lung, and Blood Institute's (NHLBI's) online calculator. https://www.nhlbi.nih.gov/health/educational/lose_wt/bmitools. htm]

DASH diet (DASH is an acronym for Dietary Approaches to Stop Hypertension) http://dashdiet.org

2008 Physical Activity Guidelines for Americans. The U.S. Department of Health and Human Services. https://health.gov/paguidelines/guidelines/summary.aspx

Lose It! - Weight Loss That Fits
www.loseit.com

Fitbit®- Fitbit.com - Find Your Fit™
www.fitbit.com/Fitness-Tracker

David Bernstein, MD is a highly respected physician who is board certified in both Internal Medicine and Geriatrics practicing in Clearwater, Florida. His 35 years of experience have provided him with opportunities to observe and empathize with thousands of adults as they age. His compassion and ability to see the souls of his patients has compelled him to share his stories in his third book *"The Power of 5: The Ultimate Formula for Longevity and Remain Youthful."* Dr. Bernstein uses 5 words that begin with the letter "S", to describe the ultimate formula he knows **can save your life**.

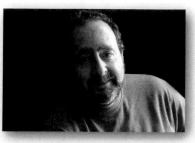

David Bernstein, MD

Dr. Bernstein is a graduate of Albany Medical College. He has served as chairman of his hospital's Pharmacy and Therapeutic committee for 20 years helping to improve patient safety and outcomes. As an associate clinical professor in the department of medicine at the University Of South Florida College Of Medicine, he has taught the skills he has acquired over the years to first and second year students.

Dr Bernstein is an avid and entertaining public speaker, addressing various medical topics with his colleagues and with the community at large with a focus on individuals and families facing the complex problems of aging and remaining healthy and youthful.

Dr Bernstein can be reached via his...
Website/Blog: www.davidbernsteinmd.com
LinkedIn: linkedin.com/in/davidbernstein2200
Facebook & Facebook Page: www.facebook.com/davidbernsteinmd
Twitter:www.twitter.com/davidbernsteinmd
Pinterest: www.pinterest.com/davidbernsteinmd

Made in United States
North Haven, CT
29 August 2022

23410418R00137